The Australian Army Medical Corps in Egypt

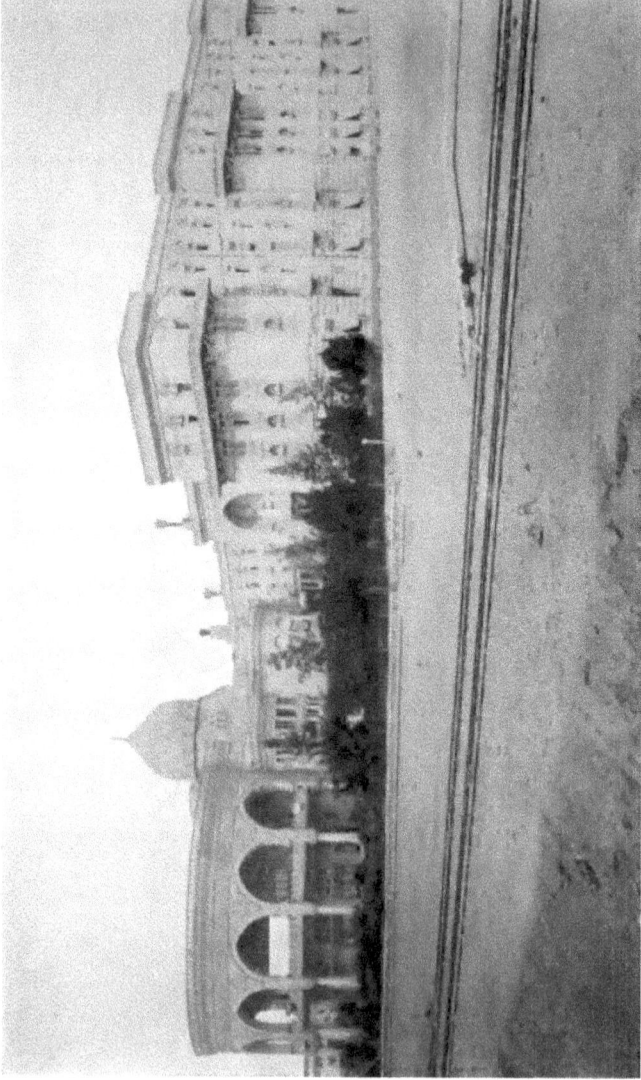

HELIOPOLIS PALACE HOTEL SHOWING ROTUNDA AND PIAZZAS

The Australian Army Medical Corps in Egypt

During the First World War

James W. Barrett
and
P. E. Deane

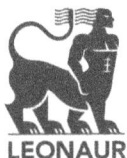

LEONAUR

The Australian Army Medical Corps in Egypt
During the First World War
by James W. Barrett and P. E. Deane

First published under the title
The Australian Army Medical Corps in Egypt

Leonaur is an imprint of Oakpast Ltd

Copyright in this form © 2013 Oakpast Ltd

ISBN: 978-1-78282-106-9 (hardcover)
ISBN: 978-1-78282-107-6 (softcover)

http://www.leonaur.com

Publisher's Notes

Contents

DEDICATED TO
SIR HENRY AND LADY MACMAHON,
IN GRATEFUL RECOLLECTION
OF THE SERVICES RENDERED BY THEM
TO THE
AUSTRALIAN SICK AND WOUNDED
IN EGYPT

Introduction

The experience of the Australian Army Medical Service, since the outbreak of war, is probably unique in history. The hospitals sent out by the Australian Government were suddenly transferred from a position of anticipated idleness to a scene of intense activity, were expanded in capacity to an unprecedented extent, and probably saved the position of the entire medical service in Egypt.

The disasters following the landing at Gallipoli are now well known, and the following pages will show how well the A.A.M.C. responded to the call then made upon it.

When the facts are fully known, its achievements will be regarded as amongst the most effective and successful on the part of the Commonwealth forces.

In the following pages we have set out the problems which faced the A.A.M.C. in Egypt, regarding both Red Cross and hospital management, the necessities which forced one 520-bed hospital to expand to a capacity of approximately 10,500 beds, and the manner in which the work was done.

The experience gained during this critical period enables us to indicate a policy the adoption of which will enable similar undertakings in future to be developed with less difficulty.

We desire to acknowledge gratefully the permission to publish documents granted by General Sir William Birdwood and Dr. Ruffer of Alexandria, and also much valuable help given by Mr. Howard D'Egville.

The beautiful photographs which are reproduced were mostly taken by Private Frank Tate, to whom our best thanks are due.

In any reference to the work of the Australian Army Medical Corps in Egypt it must never be forgotten that the expansion of No. 1 Australian General Hospital was effected under the personal direction of the officer commanding, Lieut.-Colonel Ramsay Smith, who was responsible for a development probably unequalled in the history of medicine.

The story told is the outcome of our personal experience and consequently relates largely to No. 1 Australian General Hospital, with which we were both connected.

CHAPTER 1

The Australian Army Medical Corps at the Outbreak of War

Prior to the outbreak of war in August 1914, the Australian Army Medical Corps consisted of one whole-time medical officer, the Director-General of Medical Services, Surgeon-General Williams, C.B., a part-time principal medical officer in each of the six States (New South Wales, Victoria, and Queensland, South Australia, Western Australia, and Tasmania), and a number of regimental officers. With the exception of the director-general, all the medical officers were engaged in civil practice, which absorbed the greater portion of their energy.

The system of compulsory military training which came into operation in 1911 was creating a new medical service, by the appointment of Area Medical Officers, whose functions were to render the necessary medical services in given areas, apart from camp work. These also were mostly men in civil practice, to whom the military service was a supplementary means of livelihood.

Camps were formed at periodical intervals for the training of the troops, the duration of the camps rarely exceeding a week. At these camps a certain number of regimental medical officers were in attendance, and were exercised in ambulance and field-dressing work.

In common with the members of other portions of the British Empire, few medical practitioners in Australia had regarded the prospect of war seriously, and in consequence the most active and influential members of the profession, with some notable exceptions, held aloof from army medical service.

In 1907, however, owing to the representations of Surgeon-General Williams, and to the obvious risk with which the empire was threatened, senior members of the profession volunteered and joined the Army Medical Reserve, so that they would be available for service in time of war. The surgeons and physicians to the principal hospitals received the rank of major in the reserve, and the assistant surgeons and assistant physicians the rank of captain. Some attempt was made to give these officers instruction by the P.M.O's, but the response was not enthusiastic, and little came of it.

At the same time there were a number of medical officers in the Australian Army Medical Corps who possessed valuable experience of war, notably the director-general, whose capacity for organisation evidenced in South Africa and elsewhere made for him a lasting reputation. The Principal Medical Officer for Victoria, Colonel Charles Ryan, had served with distinction in the war with Serbia in 1876, and in the war between Russia and Turkey in 1877. A fair number of the regimental officers had seen service in South Africa. The bulk of the medical practitioners concerned, however, had not only no knowledge of military duty, but certainly no conception whatever of military organisation and discipline; and what was still more serious, no real and adequate realisation of the extraordinary part that can be played in war by an efficient medical service by prophylaxis.

Such, then, was the position when war was declared.

The response from the people throughout Australia was, as Australians expected, practically unanimous. They determined to throw in their lot with Great Britain and do everything that was possible to aid. This determination found immediate expression in the decision of the government of Mr. Joseph Cook, endorsed later by the government of Mr. Fisher, to raise and equip a division of 18,000 men and send it to the front as fast as possible. The system of compulsory military service entails no obligation on the trainee to leave Australia, and in any event, the system having been introduced so late as 1911, the trainees were not available. The expedition consequently became a volunteer expedition from the outset. Volunteers were rapidly forthcoming, camps were established in the various States and training was actively begun.

Of the difficulty and delays consequent on the raising of such a force—of men mostly civilians, of all classes of society, without clothing, or with insufficient clothing and equipment of all kinds—little need be said. The difficulties were slowly overcome, and the force gradually became somewhat efficient. As both officers and men were learning their business together, the difficulties may well be imagined.

In fairness, however, it should be said that from the physical and from the mental point of view the material was probably the finest that could be obtained.

We are, however, only concerned here with the medical aspect of the movement. The medical establishment was modelled on that of Great Britain, and consisted of regimental medical officers and of three field ambulances. The director-general accompanied the expedition as Director of Medical Services, and Colonel Chas. Ryan, the Principal Medical Officer of the State of Victoria, accompanied the expedition as A.D.M.S. on the staff of General Bridges, the Commander of the Division. Colonel Fetherston took General Williams's place as Acting Director-General of Medical Services, and Colonel Cuscaden the place of Colonel Ryan as Principal Medical Officer of the State of Victoria.

The expedition left in October, a considerable delay having taken place owing to the necessity of finding suitable convoy, a number of German cruisers being still afloat and active. It reached Egypt without serious mishap in December, and at once encamped near the Pyramids at Mena.

There were some difficulties in transit. There was a most extensive outbreak of ptomaine poisoning on one ship, and measles, bronchitis, and pneumonia were much in evidence. The mortality was, however, small. The division on arrival settled down to hard training.

At once difficulties caused by the absence of Lines of Communication Medical Units became obvious. The amount of sickness surprised those who had not profited by previous experience. To meet the difficulty Mena House Hotel was improvised as a hospital and staffed by regimental and field ambulance officers.

At this stage, however, we can leave the division and return to the further development of medical necessities in Australia.

Steps were at once taken in Australia to raise a second division, and subsequently a third and other divisions in the same manner as the preceding. As time passed on, the unsuitability of some of the camps and the lack of medical military knowledge told their tale, and a number of serious outbreaks of disease took place. It is impossible to give accurate statistical evidence, but the Australian public seems to have been shocked that young, healthy, and well-fed men should *in camp life* have been so seriously damaged and destroyed. The causes as usual were measles, bronchitis, pneumonia, tonsillitis, and later on a serious outbreak of infective cerebro-spinal meningitis which was

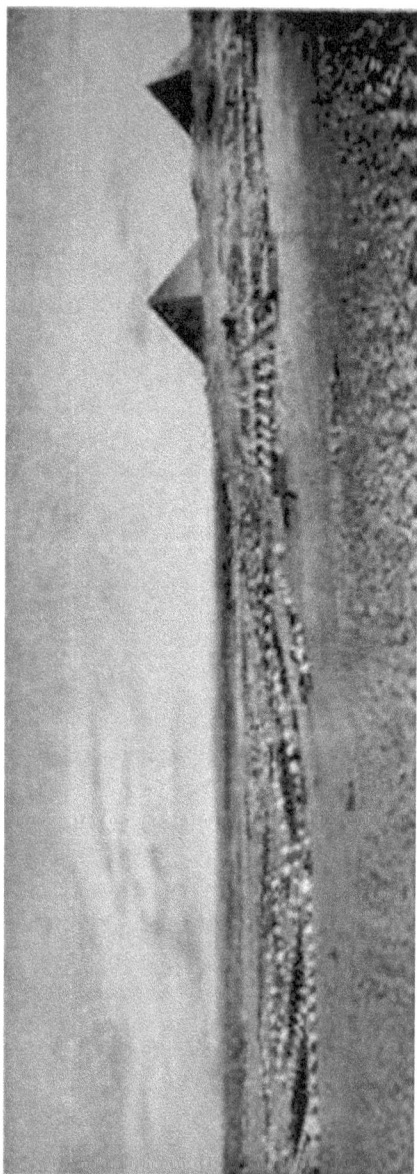

Mena Camp.

stamped out with difficulty and took toll (*inter alia*) in the shape of the lives of three medical men. The sanitation of the Broadmeadows Camp near Melbourne was not such as to provoke respect or admiration. The camp was ultimately regarded as unsuitable, and moved to Seymour, pending the necessary improvements.

It is instructive to note in passing that the Australian public received a shock when they were first informed of the amount of disease among the troops in Egypt. Yet it was apparently nothing like so great as that which existed in Australia, where the usual death-rate is so low. And yet, had the Service really profited by the lessons of the Russo-Japanese war, much of the trouble might have been avoided. The truth of course is that camp life, except under rigorous discipline as regards hygiene, and the loyal observance of that discipline by each soldier, is much more dangerous than the great majority of people seem to imagine. The benefit of the open-air life and of exercise is counteracted by the chances of infection due to crowding, defective tent ventilation, the absence of the toothbrush, and other causes.

In September, however, the Imperial Government notified the Australian Government that Lines of Communication Medical Units were required, and for the first time the majority of members of the Australian Army Medical Corps became aware of the nature of Lines of Communication Medical Units. The government decided to equip and staff a Casualty Clearing Station, then called the Clearing Hospital, two Stationary Hospitals (200 beds each), and two Base Hospitals (each 520 beds). They were organised on the R.A.M.C. pattern, and the total staff required was approximately eighty medical officers. Even at this juncture the matter was not taken very seriously, and there was some doubt as to the nature of the response. The Director of Medical Services was anxious that the base hospitals should be commanded and staffed by men of weight and experience, and accordingly a number of the senior medical consultants in the Australian cities decided to volunteer. The example was infectious and there were over-applications for the positions.

The First Casualty Clearing Station was to a great extent raised and equipped in Tasmania. The First Stationary Hospital was raised and equipped in South Australia, the Second Stationary Hospital in Western Australia, and the Second General Hospital in New South Wales. An exception to this sound territorial arrangement was, however, made in the case of the First Australian General Hospital—an exception which proved unfortunate. The commanding officer, a senior lieutenant-colonel, was resident in South Australia. The hospital itself was recruited from Queensland, but as the Queensland medical profession was hardly strong enough to supply the whole of the medical personnel, most of the consultants, including all the lieutenant-colonels, were recruited in Victoria. Now Brisbane, the capital of Queensland, is some 1,200 miles by rail from Melbourne, and Melbourne about 400 miles by rail from Adelaide, the capital of South Australia.

The result of these arrangements was that the captains and some of the majors were recruited in Queensland, together with the bulk of the rank and file and many of the nurses; whilst most of the senior medical officers, the matron, and a number of nurses were recruited in Melbourne, and the commanding officer (Lt.-Colonel Ramsay Smith) from South Australia. He brought with him some seven or eight clerks and orderlies. Furthermore a number of medical students and educated men joined in Melbourne. The bulk of the staff was, however, based in Queensland. This arrangement led to untold difficulties in the way of recruiting, and it is remarkable that the result should have been as satisfactory as it was.

The equipment was provided partly from Melbourne, partly from Brisbane, and partly from South Australia. As the commanding officer was in South Australia, as the registrar and secretary was in Melbourne, and as the orderly officer was in Brisbane, some idea of the difficulties can well be imagined—particularly when it is remembered that with the exception of the commanding officer and a few officers, the members of the staff had no experience whatsoever of military matters. Nevertheless an earnest effort was made to secure the necessary equipment and personnel. In Melbourne great trouble was taken to secure as many medical students and educated men as could possibly be obtained.

On the whole the response to the call was more than satisfactory, and Australian people were of the opinion that a stronger staff could not have been secured.

It was at first intimated that specialists were not required, but ultimately after discussion the government agreed to find the salary of one specialist. Consequently a radiographer was appointed with the rank of major, and another officer was appointed oculist to the hospital with the rank of honorary major. Subsequently he was appointed as secretary and registrar in addition, but without salary or allowances.

The equipment of the hospital was on the R.A.M.C. pattern, and was supposed to be complete. Furthermore, the Australian branch of the British Red Cross Society set aside for the use of the hospital one hundred cubic tons of Red Cross goods which were specially prepared and labelled at Government House, Melbourne.

CHAPTER 2

The Voyage of the "Kyarra"

The mode of conveyance of the hospitals to the front next engaged the attention of the authorities, and negotiations were entered into with various steamship companies. It was desirable that the hospitals should be conveyed under the protection of the regulations of the Geneva Convention.

After some negotiation and the rejection of larger and more suitable steamers, a coastal steamer, the *Kyarra*, was selected and was fitted to carry the hospital staff and equipment. The steamer is of about 7,000 tons burden. There were on board approximately 83 medical officers, 180 nurses, and about 500 rank and file, or a total of nearly 800 souls. The cargo space was supposed to be ample, and 100 tons of space were promised for the Red Cross stores.

When ready, the *Kyarra* proceeded to Brisbane and embarked a portion of the First Australian General Hospital. She then proceeded to Sydney, embarked the Second Australian General Hospital with its stores, equipment, and Red Cross goods, and then left for Melbourne, where she was to embark the remainder of the First Australian General Hospital, the First Stationary Hospital, and the Casualty Clearing Station.

On arrival at Melbourne, however, it was found that she was carrying ordinary cargo, that she was not lighted as required by the rules of the Convention, and that she was already fully loaded. Consequently the whole of the cargo was taken out of her, the ordinary cargo was removed, and she was reloaded. It was found, however, that there was no room for the Red Cross goods belonging to the First Australian General Hospital. Furthermore, a portion of the equipment which subsequently turned out to be invaluable, namely 130 extra beds donated to the hospital by a firm in Adelaide, was nearly left behind. It was only by the exercise of personal pressure that space was found for this valuable addition at the last minute. The importance of this donation will be mentioned later in the story.

Finally, after many delays, the *Kyarra* left Melbourne on December 5 amidst the goodwill and the blessings of the people, and made her way to Fremantle, there to embark the Second Australian Stationary Hospital and its equipment. She finally left Fremantle with this additional hospital, and made her way across the Indian Ocean.

Lieut.-Col. Martin, commanding officer of the No. 2 Australian General Hospital, was promoted to the rank of colonel for the voyage only. He was promoted for the purpose of placing him in command of the troopship.

The voyage of the *Kyarra* involved calls at Colombo, Aden, Suez, Port Said, and Alexandria. Those on board believed in the first instance they were proceeding to France, and when they arrived at Alexandria, and found they were all destined for Egypt, many expressed feelings of keen disappointment on the ground that they would have no work to do. They were soon, however, to be undeceived.

The voyage itself does not call for lengthy comment. The ship was unsuitable for the purpose for which she had been chartered. She was small, overcrowded, and not as clean or sanitary as she might have been. Her speed seemed to decrease, and was scarcely respectable at any time; there were apparently breakdowns of the engines; and the food supplied to the officers and nurses was not infrequently inferior in quality and in preparation. In consequence an outbreak of ptomaine poisoning took place, and twenty-two officers and others were infected, two of them seriously.

The arrangements at the men's canteen had not been fully thought out, and in the Tropics it was not possible to obtain fruit of any description. Fresh or tinned fruits were not kept in stock. There was some tinned meat and fish, but the men could obtain nothing to drink except a mixture made from Colombo limes and water.

There was a certain amount of illness apart from ptomaine poisoning, and amongst the cases treated were bronchitis, influenza, tonsillitis, and eye disease. Five cases reacted severely to anti-typhoid inoculation, and required rest in hospital.

On the whole, officers, nurses, and men took the voyage seriously, and did their best to learn something of their work. The officers were drilled, the nurses gave lessons to the orderlies, and systematic lectures were given by the officers. An electric lantern had been provided by

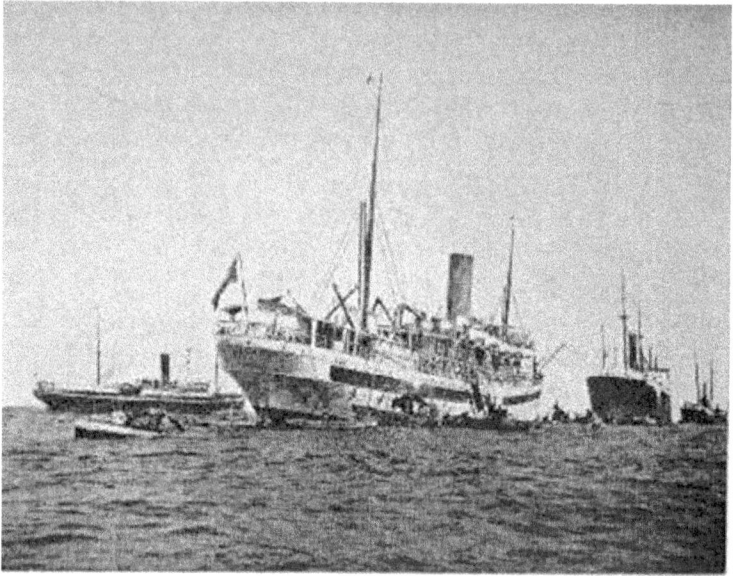

The S.S. "Kyarra."

the O.C., and lantern lectures were given regularly during the voyage.

The quarters provided in the fore part of the ship for the men were certainly insanitary, and to an extent dangerous. Towards the end of the voyage many cases of rotten potatoes were thrown overboard, having been removed from beneath the quarters occupied by the men. With Red Cross aid, however, provided by the Queensland branch, fans had been installed, and an attempt made to render these quarters more sanitary and habitable. A portion of the deck could not be used because of leaky engines, and neither request nor remonstrance enabled those concerned to get these leaks stopped.

The following measurements show what trouble so simple a fault can cause. In the tropics the wet portion of the deck could not of course be used for sleeping purposes.

APPROXIMATE DECK SPACE AVAILABLE FOR No. 1 GENERAL AND
No. 2 STATIONARY HOSPITALS

on Fore Deck

	sq. ft
Approximate deck space available	1,920
Space obtainable on hatches	288
	2,208
Space permanently wet through leaking engines	648
Approximate net	1,560

As the number of men occupying these quarters (including sergeants and warrant officers) was about 300, the space available approximated 5 sq. ft. per man.

Notwithstanding these conditions, the usual peculiarity of Anglo-Saxon human nature showed itself when at the end of the voyage the officers were required to sign the necessary certificates stating that the catering had been satisfactory. Only three refused to sign; the remainder signed, mostly with qualifications.

The manner in which the average Australian makes light of his misfortunes was strikingly illustrated on one occasion. A long, mournful procession of privates slowly walked around the deck. In front, with

21

bowed head, was a soldier in clerical garb, an open book in his hand. Immediately behind him were four solemn pall-bearers, carrying the day's meat ration, which is stated to have been "very dead." Apparently the entire ship's company acted as mourners. The procession wended its way to the stern, where an appropriate burial service was read; the ship's bugler sounded the "last post," and the remains were committed to the deep. Needless to say the usual formality of stopping the ship during the burial service was not observed on this occasion. An attempt to repeat the performance was fortunately stopped by those in authority, and all subsequent "burials" were strictly unceremonious.

Those who go to war must expect to rough it, but on a peaceful ocean, secure from the enemy, and in a modern passenger ship, it should be possible to provide food which does not imperil those who consume it, and also to ensure reasonable comfort.

With reference to the defects of the ship it should be said that when the *Kyarra* was chartered Australians had not realised the colossal nature of the war, and had not begun to think on a large scale, and those responsible had neither tradition nor experience to guide them. Furthermore the commander and officers of the *Kyarra* courteously did their best, but it was evident they understood the difficulty of transforming a coastal steamer into a Hospital Transport.

The Geneva Convention does not seem to be fully understood, and experience shows what complicated conditions arise, and how easy it is to commit an unintentional breach of the Regulations. But in war there can be no excuses.

CHAPTER 3

Arrival and Settlement in Egypt

On arrival at Alexandria, there seemed to be no great hurry in disembarking, and many of the older medical officers were fully persuaded that the units were not wanted in France; that there was very little to do in Egypt; and that if their services were not required it would be fairer to inform them of the fact, and let them go home again. They were soon to be undeceived. A message was received asking the O.C.s of the various units to visit Cairo, where they waited on Surgeon-General Ford, Director of Medical Services to the Force in Egypt. They were informed that there was more than enough work for all these Lines of Communication Medical Units in Egypt.

The First Australian General Hospital was to be placed in the Heliopolis Palace Hotel at Heliopolis. The Second Australian General Hospital was to take over Mena House and release the regimental medical officers and officers of the Field Ambulances from the hospital work they were doing. The First Stationary Hospital was to be placed with the military camp at Maadi, and the Second Australian Stationary Hospital was to go into camp at Mena and undertake the treatment of cases of venereal diseases. The First Casualty Station was temporarily lodged in Heliopolis, and then sent to Port Said to form a small hospital there in view of the imminent fighting on the Canal. These dispositions were made as soon as possible.

It should be noted at this juncture that the bulk of the Australian Forces, namely the First Division, was camped at Mena. A certain quantity of Light Horse was encamped at Maadi, whilst the Second Division, composed chiefly of New Zealanders, was encamped near Heliopolis. New Zealand had not provided any Lines of Communication Units, but her sick had been accommodated at the British Military Hospital, Citadel, Cairo, and also at the Egyptian Army Hospital,

Abbassia.

The First and Second Stationary Hospitals used their tents for the respective purposes. The Casualty Clearing Station utilised a building assigned to it in Port Said.

Some description is required, however, of the Heliopolis Palace Hotel. This, as the photograph shows, is a huge *hôtel de luxe*, consisting of a basement and four stories.

It was arranged that the kitchens, stores, and accommodation for rank and file should be placed in the basement. The first floor was allotted to offices and officers' quarters; a wing of the third floor provided accommodation for nurses, and the only portions of the building used at first for patients were the large restaurant and dining-room, and the billiard recesses, *i.e.* the Rotundas and Great Hall.

The hospital when fully developed required a large staff. The two large wards in the Rotundas and Central Hall could be administered easily enough, but the rest of the hotel consisted of rooms holding from three to six beds. The doors were removed. There were fortunately many bathrooms and lavatories. The rooms are very lofty, and provided with very large windows, but there are no fanlights over the doors, so that if doors were left in place ventilation was inadequate. A good deal of difficulty was experienced in providing suitable slop hoppers and sinks, places for cleaning bed-pans and the like, but little by little suitable arrangements were made.

The Arab servants, employed to ease the pressure on the staff, were housed in tents in one part of the grounds, and some of the rank and file in tents in another part. Others, for a short period, slept on the roof. The accommodation in general of the rank and file was excellent. The kitchens were a source of difficulty as the ranges were so elaborate; the hot-water service was unsatisfactory because of failure of fuel due to war conditions. Still, by one device and another, smooth running was ultimately secured.

When full value is given to all adverse criticism, it must be admitted that few better surgical hospitals could have been obtained.

The officer commanding the hospital (Lt.-Colonel Ramsay Smith) visited it with the registrar, and made the preliminary arrangements. He then returned to Alexandria to supervise the disembarkation. Meanwhile the registrar spent his time interviewing the proprietors, the D.M.S., and others concerned.

Only those who, knowing nothing of military organisation, tackle a job of the kind can fully appreciate the bewilderment caused by the

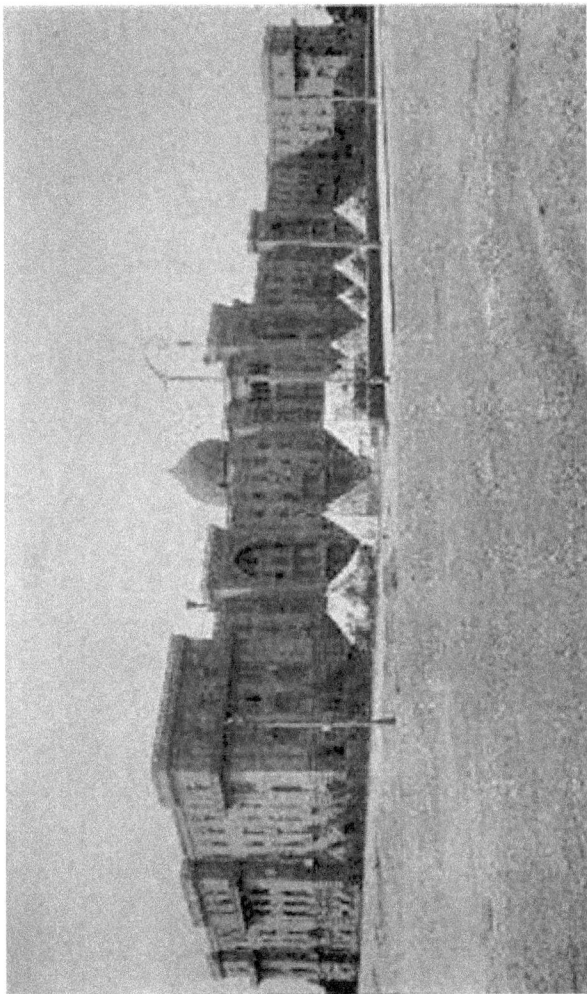

Heliopolis Palace Hotel, showing Infectious Diseases Camp.

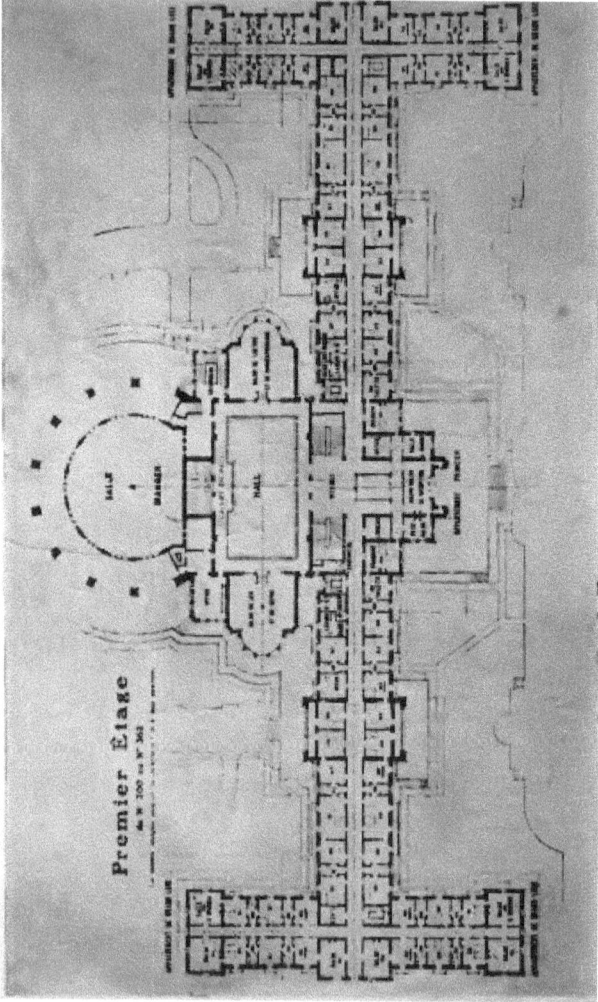

PLAN OF HELIOPOLIS PALACE HOTEL.

mystic letters A.D. of S. and T., D.A.A. and Q.M.G., and the like, with all they connote. The Imperial officers saw the difficulties and were kindly and helpful to a remarkable degree.

The hospital was opened on January 25, with provision for 200 patients. The first patient to be admitted was suffering from eye disease. An ophthalmic department was opened on the first floor, providing accommodation for out-patients as well as in-patients. As there were few oculists and aurists in Egypt at this juncture other than those at this hospital, the department rapidly assumed formidable proportions. The solid floors, lofty rooms, shuttered windows, and provision of electric light lent themselves to the creation of an excellent ophthalmic department.

The number of soldiers within easy distance of Heliopolis was not very great. Nevertheless patients, mostly medical cases, made their appearance in steadily increasing numbers, especially as Mena House was soon filled, and was limited in its accommodation.

With the arrival of the Second Australian Division in Egypt, and of subsequent reinforcements, the pressure on the First Australian General Hospital intensified, since these new arrivals went into camp at or near Heliopolis. The hotel rooms were filled with valuable furniture, including large carpets. From the outset it was arranged that neither carpets nor curtains were to be retained, and that the only hotel furniture which was to be used was beds and bedding for the officers and nurses. Everything else was stored away in various rooms. Up to this period the belief in official circles was that the First Australian General Hospital would soon be moved to France, and that it was consequently unwise to expand further, or to spend any considerable sum of money. The pressure, however, steadily continued, and when the Dardanelles campaign commenced, orders were given for the immediate expansion of the hospital to meet the ever-growing requirements of the troops. In order to effect this development the whole of the hotel furniture was moved into corridors of the building. Subsequently it was taken from the building and stored elsewhere, a difficult proceeding involving a great deal of labour.

Venereal and Infectious Diseases Camp

On February 7 a New Zealand Field Ambulance which had taken charge of the venereal cases in camp, nearly 250 in number, was summarily ordered to the Suez Canal. Orders were given on that evening at 9 p.m. that the tent equipment of the First Australian General Hos-

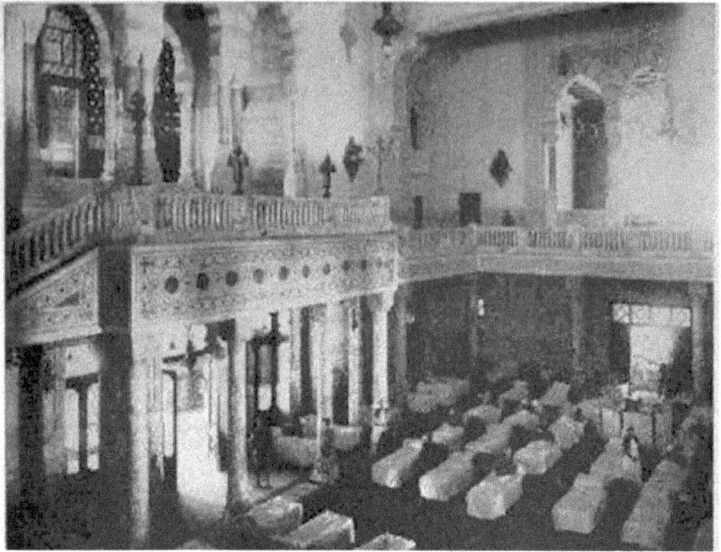

THE MAIN HALL, HELIOPOLIS PALACE HOTEL.

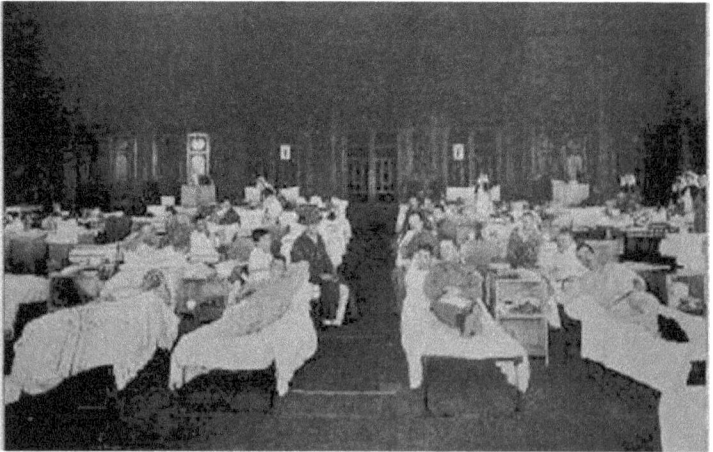

SURGICAL WARD, HELIOPOLIS PALACE HOTEL.

pital was to be erected at the Aerodrome Camp (about three-quarters of a mile distant), and that the hospital was to staff and equip a Venereal Diseases Camp by 2 p.m. the following day. By this time, too, large numbers of cases of measles had made their appearance, and it was quite clear that some provision must be made for these and other infectious cases. Accordingly another camp was pitched alongside the Venereal Camp for the accommodation of those suffering from infectious diseases. By direction of the D.M.S. Egypt, a senior surgeon was appointed to command the camp, and was given the services of two medical officers, one in connection with the venereal cases, and one in connection with the infectious cases. Definite orders were given that such cases were not to be admitted into the General Hospital.

The camp was no sooner pitched than it was filled, and the demand on the accommodation for venereal and other cases rose until upwards of 400 venereal cases, and 100 infectious cases—chiefly measles—were provided for. A good deal of difficulty was experienced in suitably providing for the serious measles cases in camp, and accordingly a limited number of tents were erected in the hospital grounds, and a small camp was formed in that position, and placed under the charge of a nursing sister. To this camp all serious cases of infectious disease, and all cases with complications, were immediately transferred. It may be said in passing that the cases treated in this way did exceedingly well.

The number of venereal cases would have wholly out-stepped the accommodation had it not been for the policy adopted by the D.M.S. Egypt. All venereal cases not likely to recover rapidly were sent back to Australia, or (on one occasion) to Malta.

Acquisition of Many Buildings

The hospital, then, at this juncture consisted of the main building, in which the accommodation was being steadily extended by the utilisation of all the rooms, and of the venereal and infectious diseases camp.

The first *khamsin*, however, which blew warned everyone concerned that patients could not be treated satisfactorily in tents in midsummer. At the request of the medical officer in charge, two rooms in one wing of the main building were given over to bad infectious cases, and the camp in the grounds was abolished. The arrangement was unsatisfactory. The cases did not do as well as might have been desired, though this was attributed to an alteration in their type; and

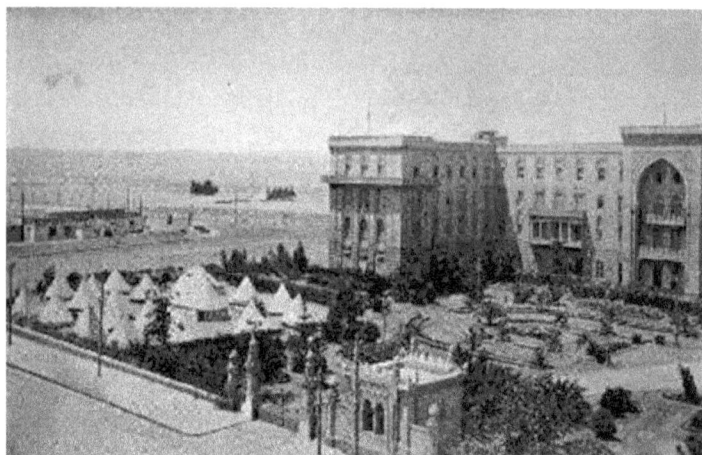

HELIOPOLIS PALACE HOTEL: ISOLATION TENTS.

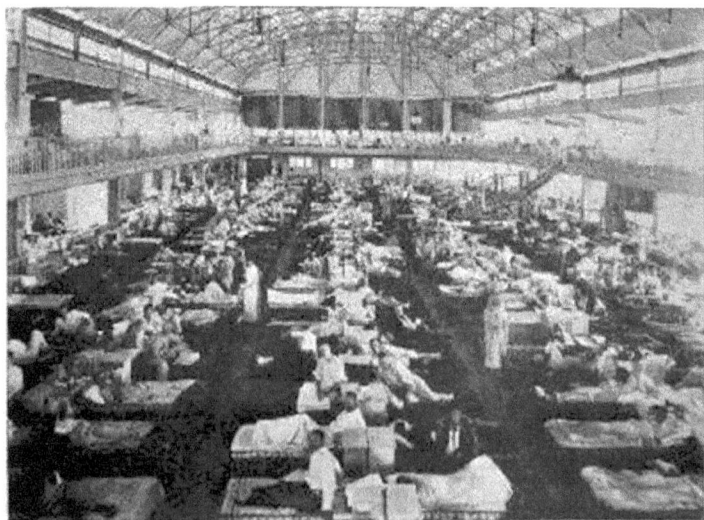

THE RINK, LUNA PARK, HELIOPOLIS.

renewed efforts were made to devise a better arrangement. Finally a portion of the Abbassia barracks was obtained, and converted into an excellent venereal diseases hospital to which the venereal cases were transferred.

The Mena camp had been struck, and the troops sent to the Dardanelles; the First and Second Stationary hospitals had moved to Mudros; and the First Casualty Clearing Station had been transferred to the Dardanelles. Consequently the pressure fell almost entirely on the First General Hospital, and the Venereal Diseases Hospital thus became the only Venereal Diseases Hospital in Egypt.

Close to the Palace Hotel there was a large pleasure resort, known as the Luna Park, at one end of which was a large wooden skating-rink, enclosed by a balcony on four sides. This building was obtained, and was railed off from the rest of Luna Park by a fence 13 feet high. The infectious cases from the camp were then transferred to it. A camp kitchen was built, and an admirable open-air infectious diseases hospital was obtained.

It became obvious, however, that the skating-rink, which with the balcony could accommodate, if necessary, 750 patients, might better serve as an overflow hospital in case of emergency, and accordingly efforts were made to obtain another infectious diseases hospital in the vicinity.

Eventually a fine building known as the Race Course Casino, a few hundred yards from the Heliopolis Palace, was obtained and converted into an infectious diseases hospital providing for the accommodation of about 200 patients. With its ample *piazzas* and excellent ventilation it formed an ideal hospital, and was reluctantly abandoned at a later date owing to the development of structural defects which threatened its stability.

The position, then, at this stage was that the First Australian General Hospital consisted of (1) the Palace Hotel, ever increasing in its accommodation as the furniture was steadily removed and space economised, its magnificent *piazzas* utilised, and tents erected in the grounds for the accommodation of the staff; of (2) the rink at Luna Park, which was now empty and ready for the reception of light cases overflowing from the Palace; of (3) the Casino next door to Luna Park, which had now become an infectious diseases hospital; and of (4) the Venereal Diseases Hospital at Abbassia, which soon became an independent command though still staffed from No. 1 General Hospital.

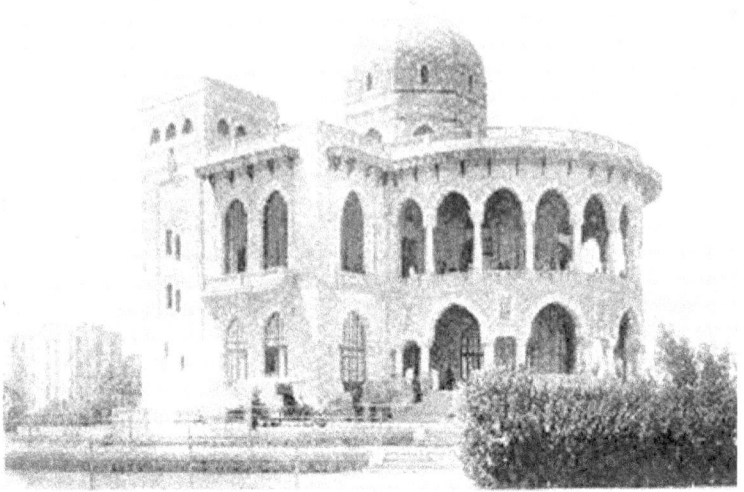

THE CASINO, HELIOPOLIS: INFECTIOUS DISEASES HOSPITAL.

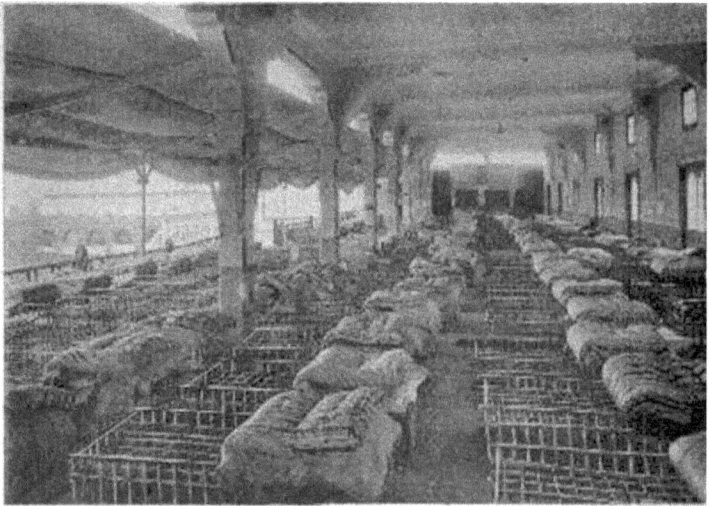

THE PAVILION, LUNA PARK, HELIOPOLIS.

At or shortly before this period, however, the authorities had become aware that wounded might be received from the Dardanelles at some future date in considerable numbers, which could not, however, be accurately estimated. Accordingly a consultation was held between Surgeon-General Ford and Surgeon-General Williams (who arrived in Egypt in February), Colonel Sellheim, who was the officer commanding the newly formed Australian Intermediate Base, the O.C. of the First Australian General Hospital, Lieut.-Col. Ramsay Smith, and Lieut.-Col. Barrett. It was decided to authorise the expenditure of a considerable sum of money in making the necessary preparation, on the ground that if the wounded did not arrive the Australian Government would justify this action, and that if the wounded did arrive a reasonable attempt would have been made to meet the difficulty. Instructions were accordingly given to buy up beds, bedding, and equipment, which would *inter alia* provide at least another 150 beds in the Infectious Diseases Hospital and 750 in the rink. At first iron beds were purchased, but it was impossible to obtain deliveries of iron beds at a rate exceeding 120 a week, and there were (practically) none readymade in Egypt. It was during this period of expansion that the donation of 130 beds made to Lieut.-Col. Ramsay Smith in Adelaide proved to be so useful.

It was, therefore, quite certain that full provision could not be made in time if iron beds were to be used, and accordingly large purchases of palm beds were made. These are very strong, stoutly constructed beds, made of palm wood. They are quite comfortable and last for several months. The drawback is that they are liable ultimately to become vermin-infected and that their sharp projecting struts are very apt to catch the dresses of those who pass by. We were able, however, to obtain them with mattresses at a rate exceeding 100 a day. They were ordered in practically unlimited numbers, so that shortly there was accommodation for the 900 patients referred to. In addition a large reserve of beds and mattresses had been created so that they could be placed in the corridors if it became necessary.

At an earlier date the project of taking the whole of Luna Park and using the upper portion of it, the pavilion, as well as the lower portion, the rink, had been under contemplation, but had been rejected on the ground of expense. The rental demanded was high, owing to the fact that the park must perforce be closed as a pleasure resort if used as a hospital.

The conveyance of sick and wounded from Cairo to Heliopolis next engaged attention, and on April 26 it was found possible to run trains from Cairo on the tram-lines to Heliopolis Palace Hotel. A trial run was made about midnight on the 27th. The first train containing sick from Mudros arrived on the evening of the 28th, and on the 29th and 30th without warning the wounded poured into Heliopolis.

As soon as the nature of the engagement at the Dardanelles became known, the D.M.S. Egypt ordered that the whole of Luna Park be taken over and immediately equipped. The pavilion was made ready for the reception of the wounded within a very few hours, and in a few days Luna Park was so equipped with baths, latrines, beds, bedding, etc., that it could accommodate 1,650 patients.

Never before in history were precautions better justified. Had the expenditure not been incurred, had the representative of the Australian Government held up the execution of the policy of preparation by waiting for instructions, a disaster would have occurred, and many wounded would have been treated in tents in the sand of the desert. Yet so strangely constituted is a minor section of humanity that instead of satisfaction being expressed that the best possible had been done, some criticism was levelled at the undertaking on the ground that it was not at the outset technically perfect, and that it showed the initial defects inseparable from rapid improvisation. The Australian people should be profoundly grateful to Surgeon-General Williams and Colonel Sellheim, whose decisive promptitude enabled the position to be saved.

CHAPTER 4

The Rush of Wounded and Rapid Expansion of Hospitals

During the first ten days of the crisis approximately 16,000 wounded men entered Egypt, of whom the greater number were sent to Cairo, and during those ten days an acute competition ensued between the supply of beds and the influx of patients. Fortunately the supply kept ahead of the demand, the pressure being eased by the immediate provision at Al Hayat, Helouan, of a convalescent hospital capable of accommodating 1,000 and in an emergency even 1,500 patients.

At the end of the ten days referred to, the position was as follows: Heliopolis Palace Hotel had expanded to 1,000 beds, Luna Park accommodated 1,650 patients, the Casino would accommodate 250, the Convalescent Hospital, Al Hayat, Helouan, was accommodating 700, and if need be could accommodate 1,500 patients, and the Venereal Diseases Hospital could receive 500 patients.

In the meantime No. 2 General Hospital had been transferred to Ghezira Palace Hotel, which was rapidly equipped, and at a later date became capable of receiving as many as 900 patients. Mena House remained an overflow hospital, bearing the same relation to No. 2 General Hospital as the Auxiliary Hospitals at Heliopolis bore to No. 1 General Hospital.

It was quite evident, however, that the accommodation was still insufficient, and a further search was made for other buildings. At this juncture a building opposite Luna Park known as the Atelier was offered by a Belgian firm for the use of the sick and wounded. It consisted of a very large brick building, with a stone floor and a lofty roof, which had been used as a joinery factory. At first the idea was entertained of creating a purely medical hospital, and of keeping the

Heliopolis Palace for heavy surgery, with the auxiliaries for lighter cases. This policy was found to be impracticable, and the Atelier was converted into a 400-bed auxiliary hospital similar in character to Luna Park.

It was open for the reception of patients on June 10, and on the 11th was practically full of wounded.

As it was evident that the accommodation was still insufficient, a further search was made, and the Sporting Club pavilion, a building in the vicinity of the Heliopolis Palace, was taken over, and converted into a hospital of 250 beds. It was at first intended to use it as an infectious diseases hospital. As, however, it possessed great possibilities of expansion if suitable hutting could be erected, another infectious diseases hospital was sought elsewhere, and wooden shelters were erected. The accommodation of the Sporting Club was raised by this means to 1,250 beds.

The heat of summer was coming on, and the necessity for providing seaside accommodation for the convalescents from Cairo became obvious. Consequently the Ras el Tin school at Alexandria was taken by No. 1 General Hospital, and turned into an excellent convalescent hospital for 500 patients. It consisted of a very large courtyard, surrounded by (mostly) one-storey buildings, and was about 400 yards from the sea. In the courtyard a Recreation Tent, provided by the British Red Cross Australian Branch, was erected by the Y.M.C.A. The whole formed an admirable seaside convalescent hospital.

But even now the accommodation was not sufficient, and by direction the Grand Hotel, Helouan, was acquired, and converted into an additional convalescent hospital for 500 patients. This institution, however, was shortly afterwards transferred to the Imperial authorities and used for British troops.

The structural defects in the Casino or Infectious Diseases Hospital, and the undesirability of using the Sporting Club for this purpose, necessitated the erection of an Infectious Diseases Hospital elsewhere. A beautifully constructed private hospital, the Austrian Hospital at Choubra, was commandeered and staffed by the First Australian General Hospital, and provided 250 beds. This hospital also was, however, soon transferred to the Imperial authorities, and administered as a British hospital.

As the demand for accommodation for infectious cases increased, the artillery barracks at Abbassia were taken over by the Australian authorities, and converted into an Infectious Diseases Hospital which

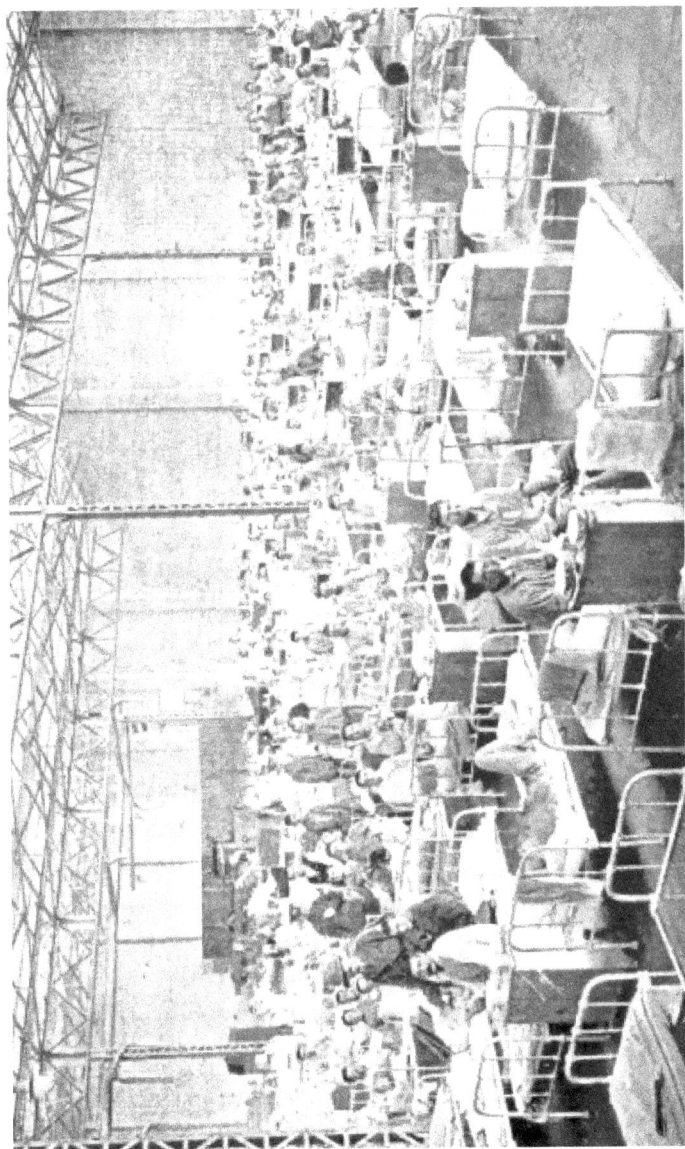

The Atelier, Heliopolis.

ultimately accommodated 1,250 patients.

The needs continuing to press, the Montazah Palace at Alexandria was offered by His Highness the Sultan to Lady Graham as a convalescent hospital. The offer was gratefully accepted by the combined British and Australian Branches of the Red Cross Society. It is the only hospital in Egypt in the administration of which the Australian Red Cross takes part.

In addition to these major activities, there were many other minor changes. The introduction of cholera from Gallipoli was feared, and in the grounds of the Casino a cholera hospital was erected in anticipated need, under the direction of the Board of Public Health, Egypt. Fortunately it was never required, but it was ready for use, and would have been staffed by the First Australian General Hospital.

The final result, then, of all these expansions was as follows. The 520-bed hospital which landed in Egypt on January 25 had expanded into:

	Beds
Heliopolis Palace Hotel	1,000
Luna Park	1,650
Atelier	450
Sporting Club	1,250
Choubra Infectious	250
Abbasia Infectious	1,250
Veneral Disease, Abbasia	2,000
Al Hayat, Helouan (Convalescent	1,250
Ras el Tin (Convalescent	500
Montazah Palace (Convalescent, Australian moiety)	500
Grand Hotel, Helouan	500
(Approximately)	10,600

Almost the whole of this work was undertaken by the staff originally intended to manage a 520-bed hospital, at all events until the latest developments. Reinforcements did not arrive until June 15, and even then they were not long available.

To house the reinforcements of nurses two other buildings were taken at Heliopolis: Gordon House, opposite Luna Park, and the Palace of Prince Ibrahim Khalim, on the outskirts of Heliopolis.

It will be noted that the greater part of the expansion took place in the immediate vicinity of the Palace Hotel. This step was alike deliberate and necessary, for reasons that will be explained hereafter.

METHODS ADOPTED IN ORGANISING HOSPITALS

The methods adopted in organising these hospitals varied. In the first instance Lieut.-Col. Barrett was deputed by the D.M.S. Egypt to seek for the necessary buildings, and when these were approved to negotiate with the owners respecting the rent. This proceeding proved very tedious and difficult, and in pursuance of a General Army Order another and simpler plan was adopted by the appointment of an arbitration commission under the chairmanship of Sir Alexander Baird. To this commission the determination of rent and compensation was referred when the acquisition of the buildings received the sanction of the commander-in-chief. It need hardly be said that a good deal of tact was necessary in these proceedings, and every attempt was made to meet the wishes of owners with regard to the buildings commandeered.

Up till June 15 the number of nurses available was small, and it became quite obvious that, owing to the rush of sick and wounded, and the hot weather, some of the nurses would experience a breakdown. Lieut.-Col. Barrett accordingly visited Alexandria, and arranged with the Australian and Egyptian branches of the British Red Cross Society to take over and equip two buildings as Rest Homes. These houses had been generously offered for this purpose to Her Excellency Lady MacMahon, wife of the High Commissioner for Egypt. One of these buildings was a large house belonging to a distinguished Egyptian and was situated in Ramleh, not very far from the beach, and the other was about eight miles from Alexandria at Aboukir Bay, the site of Nelson's victory. The latter consisted of a large seaside bungalow owned by Mr. Alderson, with an excellently fitted house-boat anchored some little distance from the shore.

The Australian Government undertook to pay for the maintenance of the nurses in these homes, which were placed under the management of a joint committee of the two branches of the Red Cross Society, under the presidency of Lady MacMahon. Nurses were then sent to these homes for a week at a time, and derived great benefit from the sea-bathing. These vacations formed a welcome and healthy break in work of excessive severity.

The following table indicates the dates of the principal changes which took place in the First Australian General Hospital.

January 14.—Arrived at Alexandria.
January 24.—Arrived at Heliopolis.
February 7.—Established Aerodrome Camp.
April 6.—Luna Park taken over.
April 19.—Established Venereal Hospital, Abbassia.
April 26.—The Casino taken over.
April 29.—Arrival of wounded.
May 1.—Prince Ibrahim Khalim's Palace taken over.
May 5.—Al Hayat Hotel taken over.
May 26.—The Atelier taken over.
May 27.—Gordon House taken over.
June 10.—Sporting Club taken over.

THE POLICY OF EXPANSION

It has frequently been said in criticism of the Auxiliary Hospitals that it would have been better to have taken over Shepheard's Hotel, or the Savoy. Neither Shepheard's nor the Savoy (particularly the former) is very suitable for hospital purposes, since hotels containing a large number of small rooms involve much labour, and consequently a large staff, and the authorities were faced with the fact that there was no staff available. Surgeon-General Williams had cabled to Australia for reinforcements long before the crisis, but the reinforcements did not arrive until the middle of June. Clearly the sound policy was to obtain buildings as close to Heliopolis as possible, to administer them with a small staff, and to use them as overflow hospitals. Shepheard's or the Savoy would have required a very large staff, and it was not existent. Even at Helouan the employment of civilians as officers was necessary in order to carry on. Arab servants were extensively employed by reason of the shortage of staff. They acted as menservants, sweepers, and the like.

MOTOR AMBULANCES

When the *Kyarra* arrived in Egypt the British authorities did not possess any motor transport. There were some motor ambulances belonging to the New Zealand authorities and a few motor ambulances which accompanied the hospitals on the *Kyarra*, and which had been allotted to special units. It became obvious, however, that units might be placed in circumstances in which they did not require their ambulances, and others in circumstances in which they required more

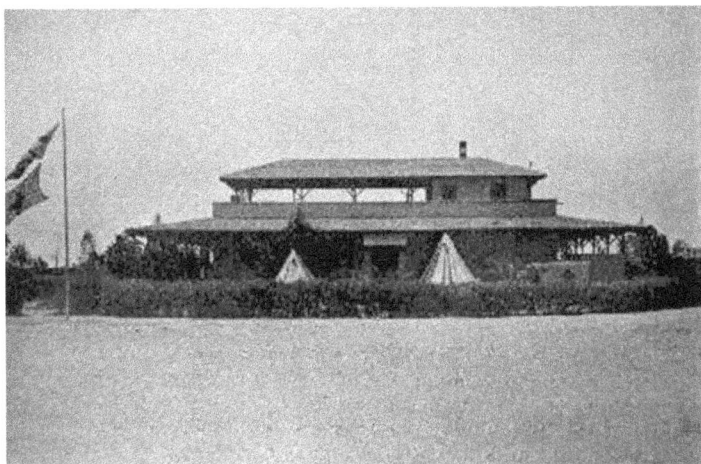

THE SPORTING CLUB, HELIOPOLIS.

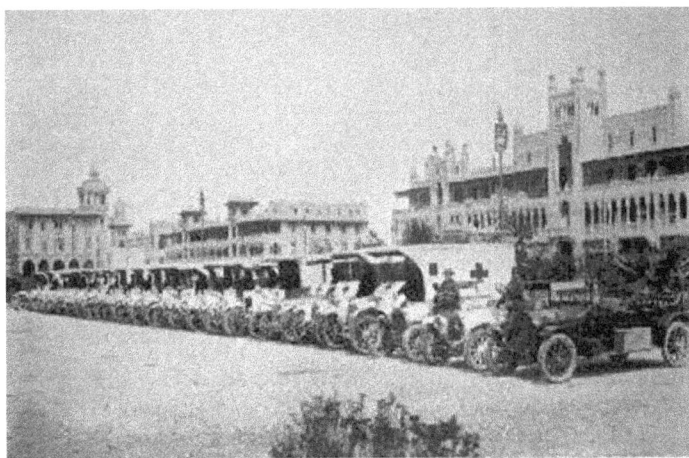

THE FLEET OF AMBULANCES, HELIOPOLIS.

than their share; and accordingly Surgeon-General Williams decided to park the whole of these motor ambulances in two garages, a major one at Heliopolis and a smaller one at Ghezira, near No. 2 General Hospital. The garage at Heliopolis held at least thirty motor ambulances. It belonged to the Heliopolis Palace Hotel, and was equipped and furnished with a repairing plant at the expense of the Australian branch of the British Red Cross. The Ghezira garage was dealt with in like manner, and in addition the rent was paid in the first instance by the Australian branch of the British Red Cross.

The organisation of these garages involved considerable difficulty. The drivers employed were not recruited by the Commonwealth Government as belonging to the motor transport, since there was not any motor ambulance establishment, and they consequently only received the ordinary private's pay. Furthermore promotions were very difficult to effect. Nevertheless they saved the position. For a long while Egypt was absolutely dependent on these motor fleets for the removal of the sick and wounded, British or Australian. The work was excessive but the drivers responded splendidly. Difficulties arose through different units endeavouring to commandeer motor ambulances for their own use. This was met by a decision of the D.M.S. Egypt that ambulances were to be kept in the garages, and telephoned for when necessary. From the outset, the lack of runabout motors was severely felt, and ambulances were frequently employed for purposes which would have been better effected by runabouts.

The Arrival of the Sick and Wounded from the Front

The end of April was reached. The bulk of the forces had disappeared from Egypt, and their position was only known by rumour; the hospital was gradually emptied of patients; Mena Camp had been abandoned, and Maadi Camp was reduced to small proportions. The weather was beautiful, and any one might have been easily lulled into a sense of false security. On April 28, however, a train-load of sick arrived. Its contents were not known until it arrived at the Heliopolis siding. The patients had come from Mudros, and numbered over 200 sick, including some 60 venereal cases, a matter of some interest in the light of subsequent events.

On the following day, however, without notice or warning of any description, wounded began to arrive in appalling numbers. On April 30 and May 1 and 2 no less than 1,352 cases were admitted at Heliopolis.

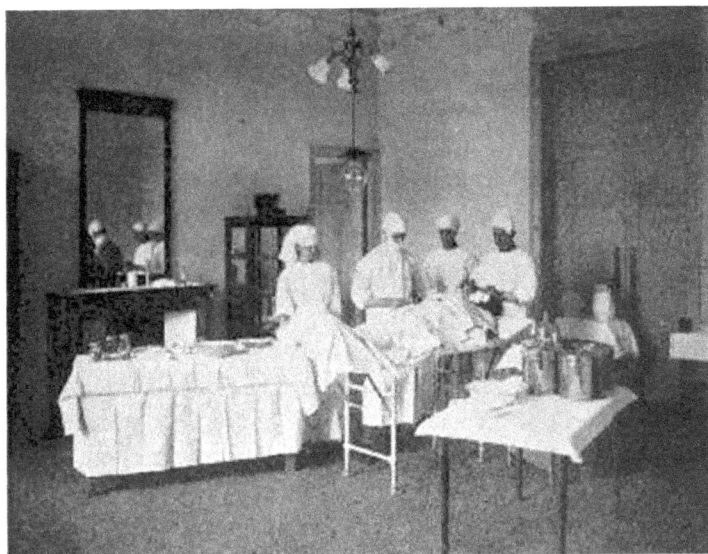

THE OPERATING ROOM, HELIOPOLIS PALACE HOTEL.

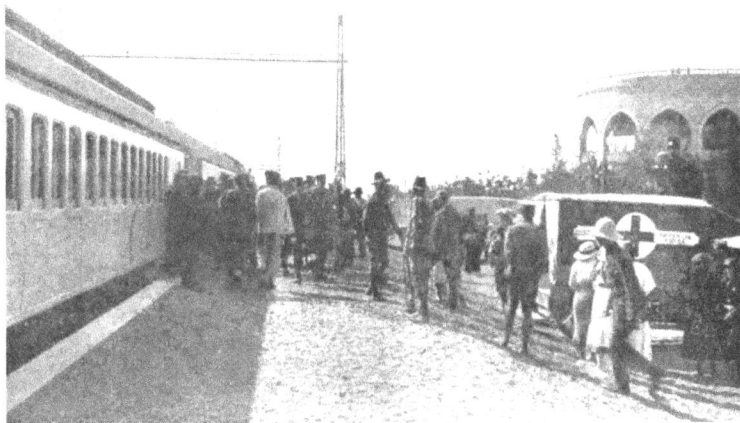

UNLOADING THE HOSPITAL TRAIN, HELIOPOLIS SIDING.

The expansion already indicated at Luna Park was at once effected, and some relief was obtained by transferring the lighter cases to Mena House—some seventeen miles distant. The last train-load of wounded arrived in the early morning of May 2, and deserves special notice, as many of the men were very seriously injured. There were about 100 cases; the train arrived at midnight, and was emptied by 4 o'clock in the morning. The bearing of the men badly injured was past praise. At 4 a.m. the main operating-room of the hospital bore eloquent testimony to the gravity of the work, which had been going on for many hours, and the exhausted condition of the staff further demonstrated what had occurred. The staff at the hospital was quite inadequate to cope with the rush, notwithstanding the willingness of everyone concerned, and accordingly volunteers from some of the Field Ambulances, and from the Light Horse units which were still in Egypt, were called for and readily obtained. With the aid of the volunteers and by dint of universal devotion to duty the work was done, and on the whole done well.

The following table shows the staff available from April 2 to August 18, and the work required of it:

STAFF, ETC., OF No. I GENERAL HOSPITAL AT HELIOPOLIS, INCLUDING AUXILIARY HOSPITALS

Date.		Officers.	Nurses.	Rank and File.	Patients.	No. of Beds.
April 25 .	.	28	92	163	495	893
26 .	.	29	92	187	504	893
27 .	.	28	92	184	479	897
28 .	.	28	92	184	479	895
29 .	.	28	92	197	631	925
30 .	.	28	92	204	1,082	1,100 [1]
May I .	.	26	92	216	1,324	1,100
2 .	.	26	92	236	1,465	
3 .	.	32	92	236	1,425	
4 .	.	28	109	221	1,427	
5 .	.	30	107	221	1,389	
6 .	.	30	107	209	1,362	2,108
7 .	.	30	107	198	1,353	
8 .	.	30	107	198	1,454	
9 .	.	29	107	201	1,432	
10 .	.	26	107	201	1,485	
11 .	.	26	107	209	1,618	2,493

[1] Including Luna Park.

44

Date.	Officers.	Nurses.	Rank and File.	Patients.	No. of Beds.
May 12 . , .	26	107	209	1,846	2,487
13 . .	28	107	249	2,293	2,592
14 . .	29	107	244	2,302	2,726
15 . .	29	107	244	2,218	2,705
16 . .	32	107	261	2,208	2,679
17 . .	30	107	259	2,165	2,646
18 . .	30	107	252	2,187	2,940
19 . .	30	107	274	1,911	
20 . .	30	107	302	1,904	
21 . .	29	107	290	1,889	
22 . .	29	107	287	1,856	
23 . .	29	107	287	1,812	
24 . .	29	104	287	1,811	
25 . .	32	104	299	1,777	
26 . .	32	104	295	1,768	
27 . .	32	104	295	1,805	
28 . .	32	104	317	1,781	
29 . .	35	143	319	1,931	
30 . .	35	143	322	1,918	
31 . .	35	143	322	1,820	
June 1 . .	35	143	322	1,876	
2 . .	35	143	315	1,873	
3 . .	36	143	314	1,869	
4 . .	36	147	277	1,866	
5 . .	35	147	277	1,872	
6 . .	36	147	264	1,786	
7 . .	36	147	264	1,627	
8 . .	34	147	253	1,709	
9 . .	34	147	253	2,474	2,805
10 . .	32	133	247	2,211	
11 . .	32	133	247	2,605	
12 . .	32	133	262	2,375	
13 . .	32	133	263	2,384	
14 . .	34	133	264	2,324	
15 . .	34	133	264	2,324	
16 . .	54[1]	171[3]	463[2]	2,269	
17 . .	54	171	463	2,328	
18 . .	55	165	462	2,259	
19 . .	55	165	449	2,266	
20 . .	55	165	443	2,339	
21 . .	55	165	439	2,335	
22 . .	55	165	439	2,357	

[1] 20 Reinforcements. [2] 38 Reinforcements.

[3] 195 Reinforcements.

Date.			Officers.	Nurses.	Rank and File.	Patients.	No. of Beds.
June	23	.	55	165	439	2,159	
	24	.	55	165	438	2,157	
	25	.	55	163	438	2,003	
	26	.	55	163	429	1,926	
	27	.	55	163	429	1,887	
	28	.	55	163	429	2,121	
	29	.	54	163	429	2,150	
	30	.	55	163	429	2,135	
July	1	.	55	163	430	2,332	2,956
	2	.	58	163	430	2,305	
	3	.	58	163	405	2,187	
	4	.	55	163	403	2,131	
	5	.	55	163	395	2,131	
	6	.	55	157	325	2,032	
	7	.	55	157	395	1,982	
	8	.	56	157	395	2,107	
	9	.	55	157	397	2,120	
	10	.	56	157	393	2,145	
	11	.	56	157	399	2,115	
	12	.	52	157	399	2,072	
	13	.	52	155	394	2,130	
	14	.	52	155	394	2,087	
	15	.	52	155	391	2,101	
	16	.	52	153	407	1,930	
	17	.	51	155	410	1,885	
	18	.	51	153	561	1,785	
	19	.	73	234	616	1,713	
	20	.	73	234	616	1,782	
	21	.	79	231	565	1,716	
	22	.	79	231	374	1,487	
	23	.	78	223	570	1,450	
	24	.	75	226	568	1,476	
	25	.	75	226	548	1,438	
	26	.	75	226	548	1,447	
	27	.	74	226	555	1,434	
	28	.	74	226	555	1,692	
	29	.	75	226	544	1,695	
	30	.	75	224	449	1,452	
	31	.	70	224	457	1,362	
Aug.	1	.	70	224	457	1,588	2,876
	2	.	70	224	457	1,610	
	3	.	71	224	447	1,652	
	4	.	71	224	447	1,631	
	5	.	61	224	447	1,759	
	6	.	60	224	456	1,731	

Date.	Officers.	Nurses.	Rank and File.	Patients.	No. of Beds.
Aug. 7 . .	60	224	456	1,793	
8 . .	60	224	424	1,927	
9 . .	59	224	432	1,902	
10 . .	58	224	432	339 [1]	
11 . .				357	
12 . .				542	
13 . .	42	216	416	454	
14 . .	47	216	462	504	
15 . .	45	216	462	535	
16 . .	45	216	480	587	
17 . .	47	216	484	485	
18 . .	48	216	460	470	

[1] Auxiliaries separated and made independent.

The proceeding adopted on arrival of the train was as follows: Two officers were on duty on the platform in control of guard and stretcher squad. The officer in charge of the train handed in a list of the number of wounded on the train, classified into lying-down and sitting-up cases, those of gravity being specially marked. The train was then emptied carriage by carriage of the sitting-up patients, who walked to the hospital or were driven by the motor ambulances as the case might be, tally being kept at the door of the carriage. As soon as the train had been emptied of the sitting-up cases, the cot patients were removed by the stretcher squad to the motor ambulances, each of which carried a load of two patients. In serious cases an officer was sent with the patient, and as the distance was less than a quarter of a mile, the transfer was fairly rapid.

The Egyptian ambulance trains were on the whole good, and were equipped with necessaries and comforts by the Australian Branch British Red Cross. The Australian military authorities also provided nurses for the trains. The stretcher squads soon learned and did their work exceedingly well; but however well the work may be done, the removal of a gravely injured man from a mattress in a wooden bunk to a stretcher offers some difficulty and may cause distress. The construction of the wooden bunks left something to be desired. There is no doubt that it is desirable to devise a carriage of such a nature that stretchers can be inserted without difficulty under every patient, and his removal effected without disturbance.

The patients on arrival in the front hall of the hospital were provided with hot chocolate and biscuits, or with lime juice, and were at once drafted to various portions of the hospital. The lighter cases were sent to the auxiliary hospitals, and the more severe cases transferred to wards in the palace building. Four sets of admitting medical officers with staffs were in readiness, and 200 patients could be disposed of in an hour. Promptitude was essential, as the trains sometimes followed on one another quickly. On admission the patients were bathed and given clean pyjamas. Their clothes and kit were sent to the Thresh Disinfector to be sterilised before being passed into the pack store.

Every patient on entering the hospital was provided with pyjamas, shirt, two handkerchiefs, socks, plate, knife, fork, spoon, mug, and slippers. The Red Cross Society provided him with writing-paper and envelopes, pencil, chocolate, nail brush, soap, cigarettes, tooth powder, and tooth brush.

As the equipment of additional beds involved the supply of all these articles, in addition to mattresses, blankets, linen, towels, kitchens, cooking-utensils, stoves, bedside tables, ward utensils, instruments, drugs, and bandages, the strain on the quartermaster's department during this period of expansion was very great. The supply and distribution of food to the auxiliary hospitals occasioned considerable difficulty at the beginning of the crisis, but was satisfactorily adjusted.

THE AUXILIARY HOSPITALS

As the patients became convalescent they were moved to one of the auxiliary hospitals, and from the auxiliary hospitals to one of the convalescent hospitals at Helouan or Alexandria, and thence either invalided or discharged to duty. As the patients during transference to the auxiliaries were conveyed in a motor ambulance, and when transferred to Helouan or Alexandria were motored to Cairo railway station under charge of a N.C.O., some idea of the work thrown on the motor ambulance corps and on the staff can be imagined.

So far all the auxiliary hospitals were regarded as wards of the main hospital, and administered from the main building—the only possible method of administration at this juncture. It was generally believed that the Dardanelles campaign would be of short duration, and that Luna Park and the other auxiliary hospitals would soon be closed. Consequently the expenditure of much money on these auxiliaries was deprecated. When, however, it became obvious that the operations at Gallipoli might last a very long time, and that in any event

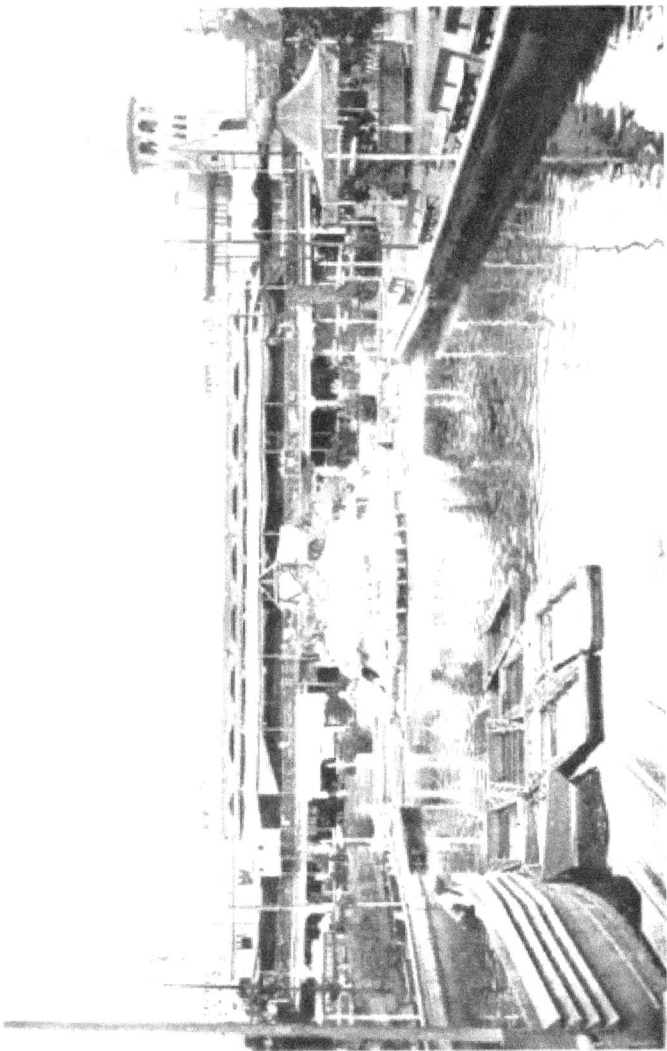

The Lake, Luna Park, Heliopolis.

the troops pouring into Egypt from Australia and elsewhere would require hospital accommodation, an entirely new view of the matter was taken, and active steps were taken to permanently equip the auxiliary hospitals for more serious work. Of this equipment something must now be said in detail.

At Luna Park the central lake was emptied and drained, and was covered by an enormous shelter shed provided by the Australian Red Cross. The shelter with a modern kitchen provided by the authorities formed the dining-room for the patients, nearly all of whom were able to leave their beds. In addition an excellent operating-room was built in brick, barbers' shops were organised, and a canteen, store, and numerous comforts in the way of blinds, sunshades, *punkahs*, were provided. Ample bath and latrine accommodation was added. As time passed, the palm beds were gradually replaced by metal beds, and the total number reduced to 1,000. In the event of another emergency, beds can be again provided, to the number of 1,650, but such a step will only be taken in the presence of necessity.

Furthermore in the case of Luna Park and the other auxiliary hospitals, the D.M.S. Egypt decided that the feeding of patients should be effected by contract, and the matter was therefore left in the hands of a well-known caterer. A large amount of Red Cross money was expended on the shelter sheds and on a recreation hut managed by the Y.M.C.A., and Luna Park became an excellent open-air hospital. It is the more necessary to draw attention to this fact by reason of the adverse criticisms which have been passed by those who have only a superficial acquaintance with it. It will be sufficient to say that up to November 1, 5,500 patients had passed through it, and there had been only one death, and that from anaesthetic. This remarkable result was not altogether due to the fact that mild cases were admitted, for latterly many major operations had been performed, for appendectomy, etc., and according to Colonel Ryan, Consulting Surgeon to the Force in Egypt, all the operation cases had healed by first intention.

In fact Luna Park really represents the triumph of the open-air method of treating patients in a rainless country. The patients preferred it because of the freedom the gardens gave them, but they showed one peculiarity which could never have been foreseen. The Australian soldier was not very fond of chairs. He did not want to stay in the shelter sheds, but preferred to spend much of his day lying in bed, and had to be ordered away from it to effect any change. It is not unnatural that men who have been doing excessive physical work should prefer

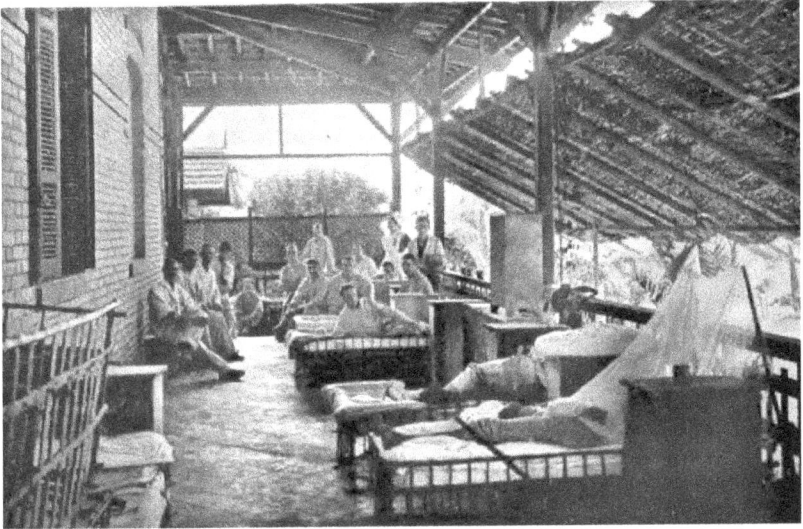

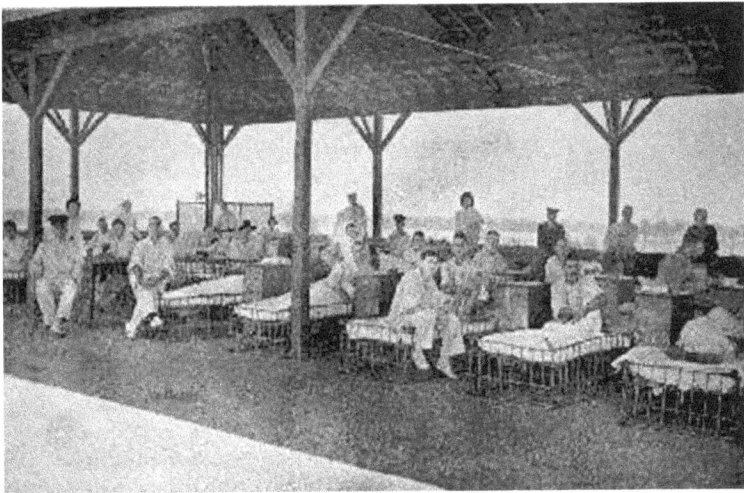

THE SPORTING CLUB, HELIOPOLIS.

physical rest when they can get it.

At No. 2 Auxiliary Hospital, the Atelier, similar changes were made. The Red Cross provided shelter sheds and a number of comforts. The Atelier was certainly the easiest of the buildings to adapt, by reason of the relatively small number of patients and its spacious surroundings.

At No. 3 Auxiliary Hospital the building could not accommodate more than 250 patients in any circumstances, but two large tennis courts were covered with matting and provided with a louvred roof. This proceeding was followed by the erection of wooden huts each of which constituted a ward of 50 beds. These huts were placed in convenient relationship to a central kitchen and other conveniences. The Sporting Club thus became an excellent outdoor hospital.

The creation of the Infectious Diseases Hospital at Abbassia is another instance of the importance of prevision. It was organised by Major Brown (who had already organised Luna Park and the Atelier) as a hospital of 250 beds. By successive squeezes, and by the erection of tents, the accommodation was rapidly increased to 1,250 beds, and was then insufficient although typhoid cases were not admitted.

The work of extension was at first difficult, but soon became quite simple because a considerable number of officers and men became experienced in the methods of effecting desirable results, and in the art of adapting means in sight to the end desired.

The Conversion of the Auxiliary Hospitals into Independent Commands

Finally it became obvious that the mechanism was becoming too complicated, *i.e.* that the administration of all these hospitals from the Palace Hotel, and the keeping of the records at the Palace Hotel, had become impossible. It was accordingly decided to separate them and make them independent commands. This arrangement was completed about the middle of August, but it involved a fresh crop of difficulties. It was quite necessary that someone should meet the trains and allot the patients to the various hospitals. That was a comparatively simple matter. It was necessary that the hospitals should be properly staffed, and that those who administered them should receive proper rank, in other words that there should be a definite establishment. This necessitated a reference to the Australian Government, and consequently difficulties and delays.

The valuable and almost essential part played by the Australian Branch British Red Cross, in effecting the expansion and in preventing a disaster, will be referred to in the chapter on the Red Cross.

The following table indicates the nature of the increasing demand on the hospital accommodation:

GROWTH OF THE HOSPITAL (FIRST AUSTRALIAN GENERAL)

Hospital opened on January 28

				Venereal and Infectious Cases
Feb.	13 .	.	186 cases	358 cases
Feb.	15 .	.	200 cases (39 Ophthalmic and aural cases)	351 ,,
Feb.	25 .	.	324 cases (including 51 special cases)	422 ,,
March	1 .	.	477 cases, 46 special cases . .	404 ,,
March	15 .	.	532 ,, 57 ,, ,, . .	476 ,,
April	1 .	.	596 ,, 64 ,, ,, . .	283 ,,
April	15 .	.	567 ,, 52 ,, ,, . .	429 ,,
April	28 .	.	479 ,, 57 ,, ,, . .	433 ,,
April	29 .	.	631 ,, 57 ,, ,, . .	478 ,,
April	30 .	.	1,082 ,, 49 ,, ,, . .	469 ,,
May	1 .	.	1,324 (286 patients discharged) .	456 ,,
May	2 .	.	1,465 (213 patients discharged) .	462 ,,
May	3 .	.	1,492	453 ,,

Patients admitted to July 31,
1915   13,325
Deaths   102=0.76 per cent.

Largest number of patients admitted on any one day
(June 8, 1915):
Australians   408
New Zealanders   85
British   325
Officers   10
                                          ———
                                              828
June 9   219
                                          ———
                        1,047 in two days
                                          ———

Sick and wounded received at the First Australian General Hospital at the end of April:

April 28   195
April 29   469

April 30	529
May 1	354
Total	1,547

Surveying in retrospect this anxious and troublesome period, the outstanding feature is the mistake made in the constant assumption that the hospital expansion was temporary. It was stated that Luna Park would only be wanted for a few weeks; the Dardanelles campaign would soon be over, Luna Park would not then be wanted, and could be closed, consequently heavy expenditure on it was deprecated. Furthermore the experience gained makes it obvious that in war the Service cannot include too many medical officers—preferably juniors. The demand for their services here and there is practically unlimited. They should be young and unattached to any particular unit—in fact a junior reserve on the spot.

It should be remembered that the expansion of No. 1 Australian General Hospital was effected under the personal direction of the officer commanding, Lieut.-Colonel Ramsay Smith, who inspected all new buildings, gave his approval or disapproval, and was responsible for their efficient equipment when converted into hospitals.

CHAPTER 5

Convalescent Depots

It will be remembered that so far as the Australian troops were concerned, provision had been made for three convalescent hospitals or homes. The magnificent hotel of Al Hayat at Helouan was taken over on May 5, emptied of hotel furniture, fitted with palm beds and mattresses, and converted into a convalescent hospital. As there was no staff in Egypt available, it was placed under the direction of a military commandant and a principal medical officer who was a civilian practitioner resident at Helouan. A few non-commissioned officers and orderlies were transferred to it from the convalescent camp in the desert at Zeitoun, which was very properly terminated.

The cooking was effected by arrangement with a professional caterer at a charge of 5*s*. a day for officers, and 3*s*. a day for men. These charges ultimately included the provision of cooking and eating utensils. This convalescent hospital both in its general character and with respect to the food supplied represents in all probability the most successful effort made in Egypt. In fact it has been suggested that the hospital was almost too attractive, and that there was consequently a good deal of disinclination to leave it. In favour of the principle involved in installing a military commandant to administer a convalescent hospital there is much to be said, as the administration is one man's work.

The Egyptian Climate

Those who know Helouan and the hotel will not be surprised at the success of the Hospital, but it may surprise even those who know Egypt to learn that Helouan is considerably cooler than Cairo, notwithstanding the fact that it is situated on the edge of the desert. Owing to dryness the Wet Bulb temperature is considerably lower than at Cairo in midsummer and the nights are always cool.

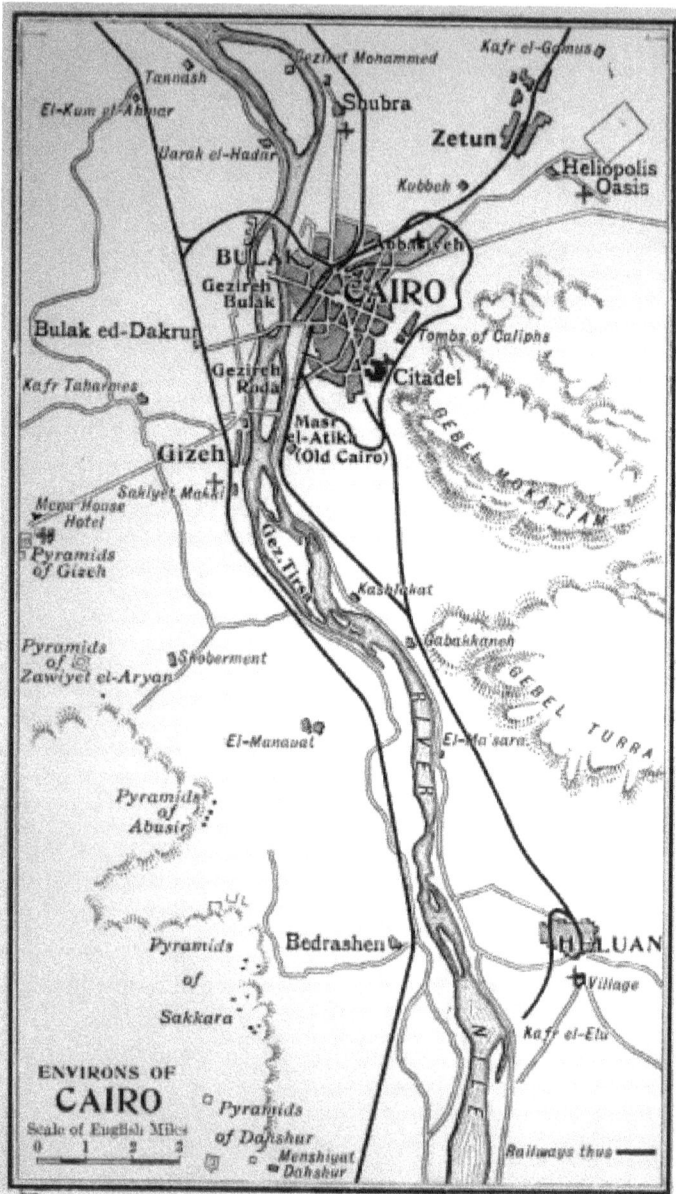

ENVIRONS OF CAIRO
The Cross indicates Medical Stations of special interest
to the Australian Force

It must be remembered that the figures in the attached table give means only, and that any registration over 75°F. Wet Bulb is high, and that at 80°F. Wet Bulb work becomes difficult. At 90°F. Wet Bulb the danger point is reached, and all work must cease on pain of death from heat apoplexy.

MONTHLY MEANS, WET BULB TEMPERATURE

	Jan.	Feb.	March	April	May	June	July	August	Sept.	Oct.	Nov.	Dec.
Alexandria . . .	53·4	54	56·5	60	64·2	71·2	73·4	73·8	69	66	61·2	56·9
Heliopolis . .	51·8	52·7	57	59·7	64·9	72·3	73	74	70·2	65·7	60·1	54·7
Helouan . .	50	50	53·8	57·4	61	67·3	68·9	69·2	68·2	62·4	57·6	52·7

Maximum at Helouan, 77·3.   Minimum at Helouan, 36·7

57

It will be seen, then, that Egypt is not especially hot, even from May till October, and that Helouan is particularly cool. These conclusions coincide with the feelings of those who live there. Alexandria is pleasant by day, because of the sea breezes, but at night most people prefer Heliopolis, which is drier and where they are more likely to enjoy a breeze.

These observations apply to the weather after May. From March to May the *khamsin* may blow for several days. The temperature then is high, but the air very dry. *Khamsins* usually cease in May.

CONVALESCENT HOSPITALS

The Ras el Tin Convalescent Hospital at Alexandria was organised on similar principles to those adopted at Al Hayat, for those who required seaside change and sea bathing. At a later period half the accommodation in the Montazah Convalescent Hospital was rendered available to Australians. The Montazah Hospital will be described under the heading of Red Cross.

By the use of these three convalescent hospitals, accommodation was provided for 1,500 patients, but in case of necessity at least another 800 could have been accommodated. In addition a large convalescent camp was erected at Zeitoun in case of emergency. After the engagement in August, a very great rush of wounded was expected, and had the hospitals and convalescent homes been really taxed the convalescent camp would have been utilised for overflow purposes. Fortunately this did not become necessary, but the experience of May had given sufficient warning of possibilities.

The normal progress, then, of a patient admitted to No. 1 General Hospital suffering from a serious wound or a serious disease of non-infectious character was removal to one of the auxiliary hospitals when he reached the semi-convalescent stage, and removal to one of the convalescent hospitals when he reached the convalescent stage. From these hospitals he was discharged to duty.

Now, Helouan is twenty miles from Cairo, and can be reached by railway or motor ambulance; and the railway station in Cairo for Helouan is eight miles from Heliopolis. As the patients were moved from Heliopolis to Helouan in scores or even hundreds at a time, some idea of the tax imposed on the motor ambulance corps can be imagined. During the crisis of May, June, and July, a visitor could witness an eternal procession of trains discharging wounded at Heliopolis, of trains discharging wounded at Cairo for other hospitals, of sick being

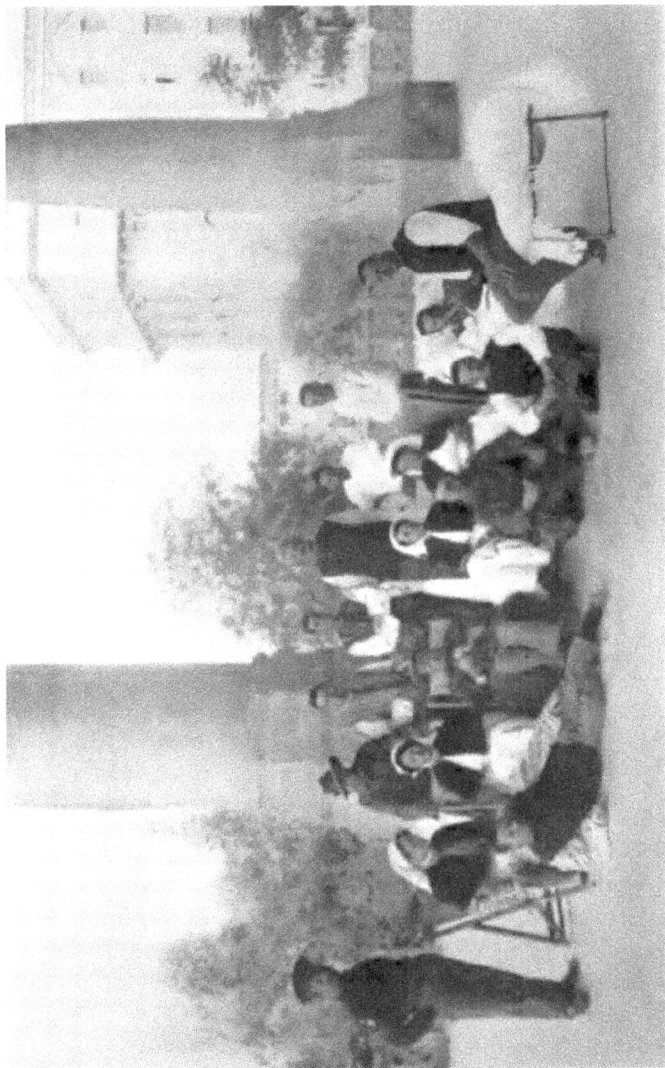

Heliopolis Palace Hotel: Convalescents on the *Piazza*.

moved to and from the different hospitals in Cairo, and convalescents from the various hospitals being sent to the Cairo station for Alexandria or to the Bab el Louk station for Helouan. Without an adequate supply of motor ambulances such an organisation would have been impossible.

It should be understood that the convalescent hospitals were available not only to all Australian sick and wounded from any hospital, but also to British or New Zealand sick and wounded. The adjustment of accounts between the separate governments was a matter of discussion, and it was finally agreed that in the case of hospitals no charges should be made by reason of the section of the force to which the sick or wounded man belonged. It was desirable as far as practicable to send the Australians to Australian hospitals, but if the treatment of the sick and wounded necessitated it, no hard-and-fast distinction was to be observed. In the case, however, of convalescent hospitals, in which the matter could be dealt with in a more leisurely way, the respective governments were charged the cost of maintenance of soldiers belonging to them.

ARMY MEDICAL ADMINISTRATION

When the *Kyarra* arrived in Egypt the military medical arrangements in that country were on a very small scale, and under the administration of the D.M.S. they rapidly enlarged. But the unexpected rush on April 29 found the British Medical Force to a considerable extent, and justly, dependent on the Australian Force for hospitals, medical officers, nurses, transport, specialists, and Red Cross stores. As there is really only one service and one object in view, it is quite unnecessary to emphasise the satisfaction felt by Australians in being of substantial service at a critical time. Since then the development of the medical services has steadily proceeded, and the anxiety of May, June, and July is never likely to be experienced again.

DISCIPLINE

A word must be said on the subject of discipline and its influence on Australians. The bravery and resourcefulness of Australians in the field are sufficiently attested by those competent to judge. Of their splendid behaviour when desperately injured we have had ample evidence, which we furnish with proper respect to brave men.

The convalescent Australian presents another problem, as also does the soldier waiting at the base. The lines in Dr. Watts's hymn come to mind. In these circumstances his very fine qualities cause him to give trouble. His ingenuity in breaking bounds is worthy of a better cause.

For example, there were complaints from the military police that sick men were roaming about Cairo at night. The roll was called at No. 1 General Hospital several times, and no one was absent. Not quite satisfied, we called the roll in the Ophthalmic Ward one evening at 8 p.m. Only one man was absent. Still suspicious, we called it again at 8.40 p.m. the same evening, and twenty-one men had gone. Some had rolled up coats or blankets and so placed them that it seemed that the men were still in bed. Subsequently uniforms that should have been in the pack store were discovered under their mattresses.

These and similar difficulties were aggravated by the fact that even a moderate disciplinarian did not always receive the support of the nurses or even the medical officers.

To illustrate: An endeavour was made to limit smoking in the wards to reasonable hours, as it has become an unfortunate tradition that a sick soldier may smoke cigarettes all day long, when in bed, without injury.

One of us (J. W. B.) entered a small ward which was filled with smoke, and was just in time to see a sick man practically blowing smoke into a nurse's face; needless to say the cigarette vanished with astonishing rapidity. Looking through the murky atmosphere, I asked the nurse whether she had seen anyone smoking, to which she un-blushingly replied, "No, sir."

If nurses and a section of officers throw their weight against en-forcement of discipline, because they don't think it necessary or right, the difficulties become considerable.

Again, the sentries were often in collusion with the men. Two in-stances suffice: A soldier got out of the hospital through a hole in the fence. On returning he determined to test the sentry with an eye to future escapades. Walking up to the gate, he said, "I want to visit a friend."

"Have you got a pass?" said the sentry.

"No," replied the sick man.

A discussion followed, and finally the sentry said, "Go in and out by the hole in the fence; it will save me a lot of trouble."

Yet another amusing incident. Sitting on the great *piazza* at Heli-opolis were a number of men convalescent from serious illness, pneu-monia and the like.

A short distance away on the outside of the iron railing fence, the

Arabs were conducting illicit and prohibited trade with the men inside, and a sentry appointed to prevent it was walking up and down studying astronomy.

The commanding officer witnessed the occurrence, visited the happy scene, interrogated the sentry, and asked him what his duties were. The sentry answered, "To walk up and down here with me gun to prevent them prisoners" (the unfortunate convalescents) "coming down them steps, and to prevent them niggers jumping the fence!"

The hardest part of military work is waiting. The soldier who has the magnificent fundamental qualities of the Australian, and who can wait and obey, would be the greatest soldier on earth. We are hopeful that the experience gained will render the Australian the claimant for this coveted position. All thoughtful Australian officers we know tell the same story: "Give us discipline, and again and again discipline."

There is much to be said for the soldier. He will obey if he knows why an order is given, or if he trusts his officer and knows why it is given. But if he is uncertain on these points he pleases himself. Discipline cannot be enforced in general, except by properly trained professional officers.

Again, there was more drunkenness than there should have been from the same cause. One evening visitors passed liquor into hospital, and a hideous din arose. On seeking the cause, I discovered it to proceed from a ward containing three patients, of whom one had a broken leg and another a broken arm.

These two men were uproariously drunk, and were sitting up in bed making Australian political speeches. On my entry he of the broken leg demanded in broken tones to be at once paraded before the orderly officer.

On another occasion a particularly nuggety patient had broken the rules, and becoming troublesome was ordered back to his ward. Refusing to go, the guard was sent for, and a fight of a desperate character ensued before he was overpowered; yet we found accidentally that later on this man was made a N.C.O. and apparently gave satisfaction.

In other armies such an offence might have been punished with death.

On reading the account of the life of Stonewall Jackson it is clear that similar difficulties were experienced with the Confederate soldiers, and that Jackson against his inclination was compelled to enforce grave penalties at times to prevent still graver trouble.

It takes several men on the lines of communication and at the base to keep one man at the front, and only loyal obedience to orders during the wearisome and exacting day's work on the lines of communication will make the machine run smoothly, and do justice to the man in the line of battle who is risking his life.

Yet it seems to us there is much to be done by attention to the soldiers' social wants. The work of the Y.M.C.A. and the provision of soldiers' clubs were powerful influences in favour of good order and conduct.

CHAPTER 6

Evacuation of the Unfit

It became evident, both during the crisis and before the expected attack in August, that Egypt must be cleared of those who were not likely to be fit for service in the immediate future. The necessary effort made to send invalids away for change, and to send the permanently disabled home, involved important questions of policy the determination of which took time. A number of problems at once obtruded themselves. Who was to be permanently invalided, and how was the determination to be reached? Who was to be sent away temporarily, and for how long was he to go? Where was he to be sent to? What was to be done with malingerers, of whom there was a small but sufficiently numerous percentage? As regards the first question: is a man, for example, who has lost an eye permanently invalided? Is he fit for base duty in Egypt, or must he be sent home?

It is hardly fair to send him to the front and expose him to the risk of total blindness. In this particular case, in view of the possibilities of the development of ophthalmia in Egypt—which, by the way, did not prove nearly as serious as was anticipated—it was decided that the man who had lost one eye should be sent home as permanently unfit. Men who had lost a limb were put in the same category. It might be argued that such men were quite fit for clerical work, and that one-eyed men were quite fit for ordinary guard work, for which, indeed, the demand was overwhelming. The view already indicated, however, was taken, and these men were sent to their homes to be discharged. But when these definite and obvious cases were disposed of, there remained some thousands of men whose cases were full of difficulty. In each hospital boards were accordingly appointed to investigate their cases and to fully answer the questions set out in the following Army Form B 179.

MEDICAL REPORT ON AN INVALID
(TAKEN FROM ARMY FORM B 179)
8. Disability
Statement of Case
Note.—*The answers to the following questions are to be filled in by the officer in medical charge of the case. In answering them he will carefully discriminate between the man's unsupported statements and evidence recorded in his military and medical documents. He will also carefully distinguish cases entirely due to venereal disease.*

9. Date of origin of disability.

10. Place of origin of disability.

11. Give concisely the essential facts of the history of the disability, noting entries on the Medical History Sheet bearing on the case.

12. (*a*) Give your opinion as to the causation of the disability.

(*b*) If you consider it to have been caused by active service, climate, or ordinary military service, explain the specific conditions to which you attribute it. (*See* Notes.)

13. What is his present condition?
Weight should be given in all cases when it is likely to afford evidence of the progress of the disability.

14. If the disability is an injury, was it caused—
   (*a*) In action?
   (*b*) On field service?
   (*c*) On duty?
   d) Off duty?

15. Was a Court of Inquiry held on the injury?
If so—(*a*) When?
   (*b*) Where?
   (*c*) Opinion?

16. Was an operation performed? If so, what?

17. If not, was an operation advised and declined?

18. *In case of loss or decay of teeth.* Is the loss of teeth the result of wounds, injury, or disease, directly[1] attributable to active service?

19. Do you recommend—
   (*a*) Discharge as permanently unfit, or
   (*b*) Change to England?

---

1. Loss of teeth on, or immediately after, active service, should be attributed thereto, unless there is evidence that it is due to some other cause.

....
Officer in medical charge of case.
I have satisfied myself of the general accuracy of this report, and concur therewith, *except* [2]

Station. . . . .
Officer in charge of Hospital.
Date. . . . .

OPINION OF THE MEDICAL BOARD

Notes.—(*1*) Clear and decisive answers to the following questions are to be carefully filled in by the Board, as, in the event of the man being invalided, it is essential that the Commissioners of Chelsea Hospital should be in possession of the most reliable information to <u>enable them to decide upon the man's claim to pension</u>.

(2) Expressions such as "may," "might," "probably," etc., should be avoided.

(3) The rates of pension vary directly according to whether the disability is attributed to (*a*) active service, (*b*) climate, or (*c*) ordinary military service. It is therefore essential when assigning the cause of the disability to differentiate between them (*see* Articles 1162 and 1165, Pay Warrant, 1913).

(4) In answering question 20 the Board should be careful to discriminate between disease resulting from military conditions and disease to which the soldier would have been equally liable in civil life.

(5) A disability is to be regarded as due to climate when it is caused by military service abroad in climates where there is a special liability to contract the disease.

20. (*a*) State whether the disability is the result of (1) active service, (2 climate, or (3) ordinary military service.

(*b*) If due to one of these causes, to what specific conditions do the Board attribute it?

21. Has the disability been aggravated by—

(*a*) Intemperance?

(*b*) Misconduct?

22. Is the disability permanent?

23. If not permanent, what is its probable minimum duration? *To be stated in months.*

---

2. Delete this word if no exceptions are to be made.

24. To what extent is his capacity for earning a full livelihood in the general labour market lessened at present?
In defining the extent of his inability to earn a livelihood, estimate it at ¼, ½, ¾, or total incapacity.

25. If an operation was advised and declined, was the refusal unreasonable?

26. Do the Board recommend—

    (*a*) Discharge as permanently unfit, or

    (*b*) Change to England?

Signatures:—

                                  . . . . *President.*

                              . . . .

Station. . . . .   *Members.*

Date . . . .

      Approved.

Station . . . .

                               Administrative Medical Officer.

Date . . . .

It should be remembered that the bulk of the medical officers were civilians, that they were unaware of the broad questions of policy involved, and that they were inclined on principle to give a holiday to a man who had been fighting, and even to believe the stories told them by the malingerer. The reader will therefore not be surprised to learn that a number of men who were certainly not in a very bad way were recommended for two, three, or six months' change, or even for discharge. The proceedings of the board were reviewed by a responsible officer; for a long time by Lieut.-Col. Barrett when acting as A.D.M.S. on General Ford's staff. It was, however, difficult to persuade any board which had once expressed their opinion to modify it, and almost impossible to get them to reverse it. If their recommendations had been rejected altogether, the conduct of the service would have become difficult. Under direction, an attempt was made to modify the practice by appointing a permanent board in each hospital, presided over by a senior medical officer charged with the duty primarily of attending to Board work, and of acting as a clinician only when he had time.

THE FOLLOWING DRAFT WAS MADE THE BASIS
OF THE ARRANGEMENT

1. Two medical officers are to be detached from other duties at Nos. 1 and 2 Australian General Hospitals respectively, in order to form a

majority of a permanent invaliding board at each hospital. They will be known as the senior and junior invaliding officer respectively.

2. The duties of the Board at Nos. 1 and 2 Australian General Hospitals will be to form an Invaliding Board by meeting in each case the medical officer in charge of the case.

3. The Board proceedings when completed will be sent to the A.D.M.S. Australian Force, Headquarters, Cairo, and on being approved will at once be forwarded with nominal roll to the Australian Intermediate Base Depot, Cairo.

4. The Australian Intermediate Base will forward to the O.C. Hospital or Convalescent Home nominal roll of patients who are to be discharged or transferred to Australia or England. These patients will be transferred to the Convalescent Home, Helouan (if they are able to leave hospital), and will remain at the Home till transport is ready for them.

5. The only circumstances in which completed Board cases are to be retained in any hospital, except the Convalescent Home, Helouan, are when patients require a considerable amount of treatment, and are unfit to leave the hospital.

6. The senior invaliding officer will be responsible for the accuracy of the nominal rolls.

7. At Alexandria an invaliding officer will be attached to the Australian Convalescent Home at Ras el Tin. It will be his duty, under direction of the A.D.M.S. Alexandria, to proceed to the various hospitals and camps in Alexandria, arrange for the formation of Boards, of which he will be a member, to deal with all cases in Alexandria. These cases, in like manner, must be forwarded to Convalescent Home, Helouan, except in the cases of those who are unfit to leave hospital.

8. The cases to be dealt with fall into two classes: (*a*) men unfit for military service, who may be sent by (1) transport to Australia or (2) by hospital ship to Australia; and (*b*) men likely to profit by change to England during hot weather, to proceed by (1) transport or (2) hospital ship.

9. The Board proceedings are to indicate, in the opinion of the Board, the best manner of dealing with patients under the several headings.

June 30, 1915.

Again difficulties arose, since none of the medical officers wanted the job. In fact, medical officers in general never want to do anything except attend to patients. They are unsuited temperamentally for administrative work, and dislike it. Even with this modification, though the system worked somewhat better, evils obtruded themselves. The statements of men who swore they were suffering from rheumatism and severe pains in the back were sometimes taken at face value, and further modification consequently became necessary. Any medical officer could recommend any patient to be boarded. The Board then sat and sent in its report to the A.D.M.S. Under the modified arrangement no patient could be boarded until he had been examined by the senior medical officer of the Australian Force in Egypt, or by the D.D.M.S. Egypt, Col. Manifold. By this means most of the trouble was eliminated and a satisfactory principle was established. It is the old story—the reversion to direction by a limited number of experienced and responsible people.

It was decided not to send Australian patients to Great Britain other than in exceptional cases, that is if they had friends or relatives there, and if they only required a short change, say two months. As the voyage to Australia occupied a month each way, it was absurd to send them back there for two months. For three months or more they were sent to Australia, and in some cases were discharged on arrival. Some men who were no longer fit for service at the front were kept in Egypt for Base Duty.

Only those who have experience of base work become aware of the enormous demands made on a garrison for guard work, for clerical work, orderly work, and the like. At Al Hayat, Helouan, for example, the commandant really required ninety men for sentry work, though he had only forty. The demands for competent clerks were incessant.

As soon as patients were destined for dispatch to Australia they were forwarded to Helouan and kept there until the ship was ready to leave. As a result Helouan was filled with waiting cases. In order then to ease the pressure at Helouan, a waiting camp was established at Suez close to the Government Hospital, to which any patients could be admitted. This establishment of course necessitated further demands for medical officers, orderlies, etc.

Transport of Sick and Wounded by Sea

As soon as it was decided to return patients to Australia in addition to those sent to England, Cyprus, or convalescent hospitals in Egypt, a system was developed in order to provide the necessary staffs and equipment on ships. Surgeon-General Williams had exerted himself

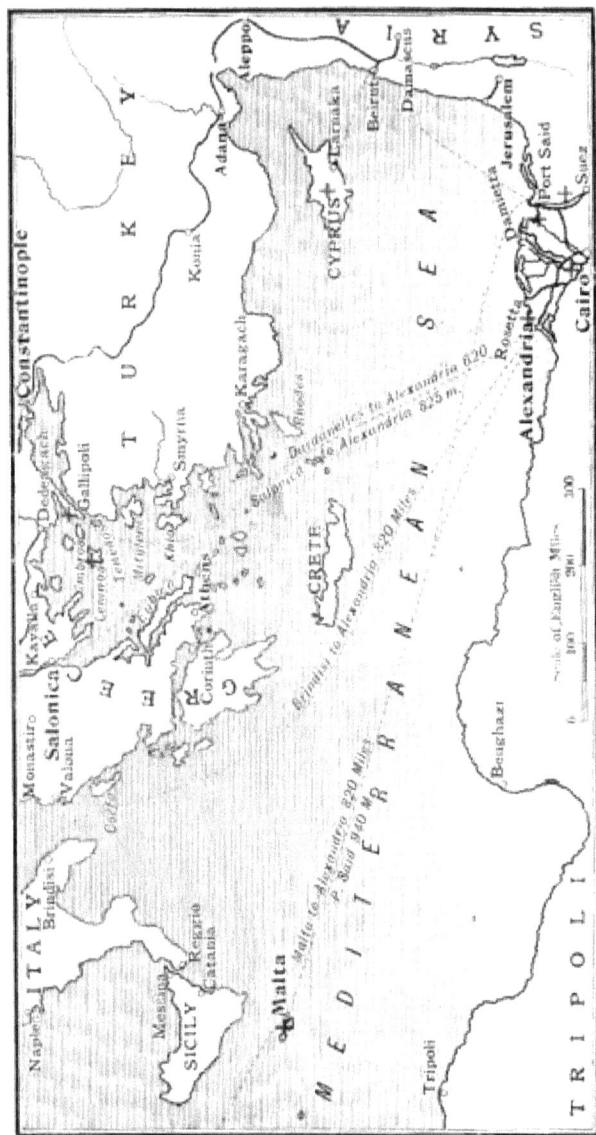

THE EASTERN MEDITERRANEAN.

The Cross indicates Medical Stations of special interest to the Australian Force.

to get hospital ships provided, but in the early stages they had not even been promised, and a service was perforce created by utilising empty transports and collecting the staff in Egypt. The first efforts may be described as almost maddening. It was impossible to get adequate notice when a ship was likely to leave for Australia. It had probably been to the Dardanelles and unloaded soldiers and munitions of war. It had returned to Alexandria packed with wounded. It might then be drafted to Australia, at a few days' notice. It was necessary to clean and refit it, to place hammocks, blankets, beds on board, to provide drugs and surgical appliances and Red Cross stores, and to provide a staff in Egypt.

In looking back on the efforts made, the wonder is not that minor defects occurred in the early stages, but that the work was done anything like as well as it was. The difficulties were almost insuperable, and nothing but the devotion of a number of medical officers to the service rendered any decent result possible.

The first ship to leave with wounded on board was the *Kyarra* on June 7, but previously a number of ships had left containing invalids, venereal cases, undesirables, and oddments. In every case there was a scramble at the last moment to get things ready. The staff for the ships was provided by detailing officers, nurses, and orderlies from the scanty staffs of Nos. 1 and 2 General Hospitals. The Australian Government, under request, then began to provide transport staffs who came with the troopships and returned at later intervals when the troopships went back again as "hospital carriers." Of hospital ships proper there were none.

Each ship was inspected in order to ascertain the number of patients she could carry, and to determine the staff requisite—consequently a routine procedure was adopted. Cot cases were seldom taken, as it was thought better where possible to keep cot cases in Egypt. A minimum of two medical officers was allowed for 300 patients, and an additional medical officer for every 150 patients. One trained nurse was allowed for every 50 patients, and one orderly for every 25 patients. These numbers were arbitrary and approximate, but served as a working basis. The supply was probably in excess of real requirements, but it was necessary to contemplate the possibility of an epidemic outbreak in the tropics and the grave results which might ensue. The equipment of drugs and instruments was liberal, and was arranged on a fixed plan worked out by the officer in charge of the base medical store at Heliopolis. The Red Cross stores were supplied in the same way, and the commanding officer was given a sum of money, sometimes as much as £150 to £200, to spend on comforts for the men. A canteen was placed on board in addition. The ship was not allowed to leave the wharf until the commander had given a certificate that he had on board all the medical comforts required by the Admiralty regulations, and until the principal medical officer had given a certificate that he had all that he required in the way of staff, drugs, surgical and medical equipment, and Red Cross stores.

There is no more dangerous branch of medical service than the transport of sick and wounded over the ocean, since there are so many possibilities of disaster.

Base Medical Store

These continual demands on personnel and on medical stores necessitated suitable arrangements, and messages were sent to Australia asking for reinforcements. In addition a large base medical store was established at Heliopolis, and made an independent unit. It became the business of the officer in charge of this store, Captain Johnson, to make up drugs and surgical instruments per 100 patients, and to receive the surplus stores from each of the incoming transports. Two hospital ships were ultimately provided, the *Karoola* and the *Kanowna*, and reached Egypt in October.

Transport of Sick and Wounded to Suez

The arrangements for conveying the invalids from Cairo to Suez were interesting. They could not be conveyed to Alexandria or Port Said because one passenger placed on a ship at those ports enormously increased the charges made by the Suez Canal Company, and Suez was consequently fixed upon as the port of departure and the port of equipment. Patients to be conveyed to Suez were at Helouan, or at different hospitals in Cairo, and accordingly two trains were made up—one at Helouan and one at Palais de Koubbeh, Heliopolis. Each train was filled at a specific time, the two trains conveyed to Cairo, a junction effected in the Cairo station, and the whole conveyed to Suez. The journey took about five hours, and the necessary provision was made for feeding the men on the way. One of the difficulties in conveying such patients was to prevent them riding on the platforms of the carriages and falling off. A sentry was placed at each end of the carriage to prevent the continuance of these disasters, which had been too numerous in the case of healthy men in the troop trains. Men

CASES RETURNED TO AUSTRALIA FROM FEB. 3 TO SEPT. 25, 1915, AND REASONS

Officers = O.   Other ranks = O. R.

Medically Unfit.		Venereal Cases.		Services no longer required.		Other Reasons.		Change to Australia.		Total.		Wounded in Action.	
O.	O.R.	O.	O.R.	O.	O.R.	O.	O.R.	O.	O.R.	O.	O.R.	O.	O.R.
29	2,496	450 also sent to Malta	1,344	5	215	24	49	29	1,154	137	5,258	52	1,571

73

had even lost their lives or been mutilated from trying to ride on the buffers *à la Blondin*.

On arrival at Suez the train proceeded alongside the ship, the patients and their kit were moved on board, and a guard placed in the dockyard. Even then men straggled into Suez, and their recapture gave some trouble. The Australian is essentially a roamer.

The table on the previous page indicates the number of soldiers returned to Australia up to September 25, 1915, and the reason for their transfer.

THE CROSS INDICATES MEDICAL STATIONS OF SPECIAL INTEREST TO THE AUSTRALIAN FORCE.

CHAPTER 7

Sickness and Mortality Amongst Australians

In civil practice we had long been aware of the fundamental failing of the medical profession. Its members operate in a community as individuals. They seek to cure disease in general; they are conscientious to a degree in the discharge of this duty, and they give valuable personal advice respecting hygiene. But of the prophylaxis of disease they have little trained knowledge, and they are not seriously interested. The prophylaxis of disease really implies organised and co-operative effort, and can only be effectively undertaken by those public-health officials who are charged with it as a definite function. In Australia at all events the inducements to enter the public-health service as a profession are not very great. The influence of the department is not very far-reaching, and the prophylaxis of disease is still in its infancy. One can foresee the time when the number of practitioners per 100,000 of the population will be fewer than at present, and the number of public-health officials will be greater. The transition from the one occupation to the other will only take place when a much higher standard of general intelligence prevails in the community.

What applies to civil life applies to a lesser extent to an army, because the headquarters staff of an army are as a rule excellently informed respecting the risk run by neglect of sanitation. They understand thoroughly that disease may do more harm than battles, and that outbreaks permitted to get out of hand are with difficulty controlled. In the Australian Army, by reason of its necessarily scratch nature, there was practically no instruction in prophylaxis. It was certainly not acutely understood, and the disastrous events which attended the formation of camps in Victoria and elsewhere show that the controlling authorities were either not fully informed of the risks, or if informed, did not understand the best plan of action. What applied in Australia was true to a lesser extent in Egypt, because Surgeon-General Williams and many of the R.A.M.C. officers who controlled medical operations in Egypt, and distinguished members of the Indian Medical Service who were associated with them, had been through a number of campaigns in South Africa and elsewhere, and were aware both of the risks and the difficulties. Consequently some effort was made to avoid, or to minimise the effects of, some of the disastrous outbreaks.

In March and April, before the arrival of wounded, the number of cases in hospital was a source of common comment amongst the medical officers, who could not understand why healthy men under service conditions, camped on the edge of a dry desert, should be suffering from serious disease to such an extent. The diseases were for the most part measles, with its complications, bronchitis, broncho-pneumonia, and a certain amount of lobar pneumonia, infectious pleuro-pneumonia, and tonsillitis. There were a few cases of cerebro-spinal meningitis. The impression made on a physician who had all the cases coming from the Heliopolis camps under his control was that these diseases were inordinately prevalent; but the following figures, obtained from headquarters and forwarded to the government, show that while disease was more extensive than it should be, it was not excessive. Including venereal disease, the cases certainly did not exceed 6 to 8 *per cent.* of the force.

FIRST AUSTRALIAN GENERAL HOSPITAL

Memorandum prepared to show the Extent of Disease amongst Australian Troops

Palace Hotel,
Heliopolis,
May 8, 1915.

(Report begins)

The following figures have been obtained from the office of the D.M.S. Egypt. Owing to the movement of troops out of Egypt, comparisons are apt to be a little difficult to institute with accuracy. Nevertheless the figures given substantially indicate the position.

On February 15 there were 1,329 patients in hospital. The number of sick and off duty in the lines, but not in hospital, is not stated; but as it amounted to 423 on February 1, and to

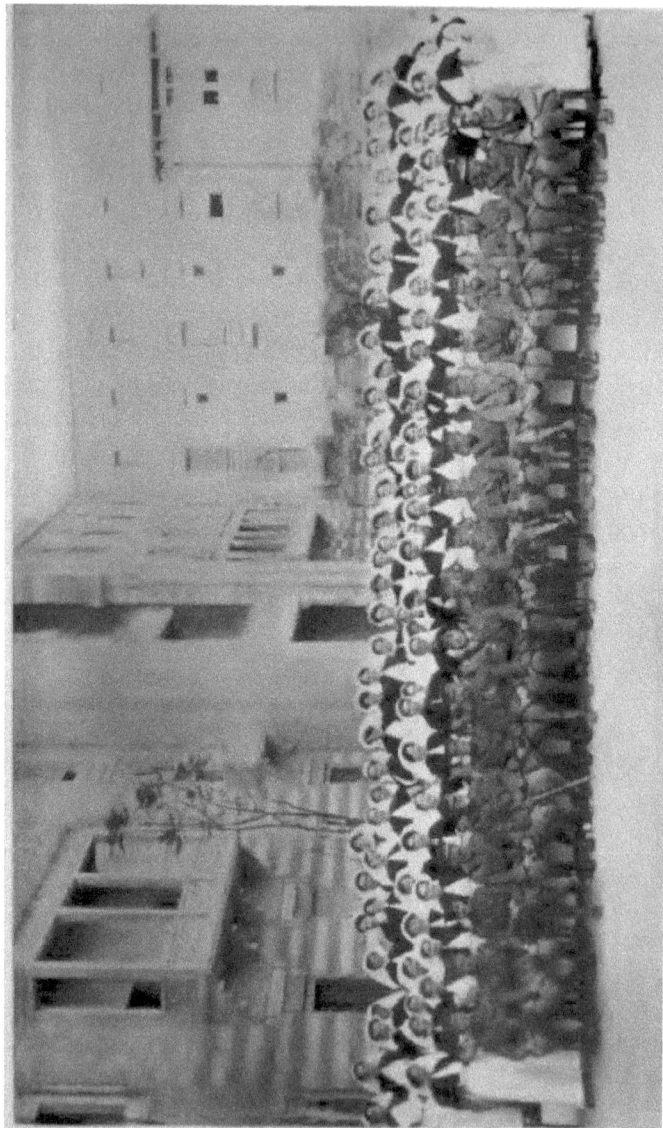

Officers and Nurses, No. 1 Australian General Hospital.

644 on March 1, it may be assumed to be 500, which will give a total of 1,829 sick and off duty on February 15.

On March 1, 1,737 men were in hospital, 644 off duty and sick in the lines, or a total of 2,361.

On March 15, 1,429 were in hospital, 500 off duty and sick in the lines, or a total of 1,929.

On April 1, 1,217 were in hospital, 495 sick and off duty in the lines, or a total of 1,712.

The totals, therefore, off duty on the dates specified were:

February 15 (approx.)	1,829
March 1	2,381
March 15 (approx.)	1,929
April 1	1,712

It should be stated that the figures quoted above would have been very much larger were it not that a large number of men unfit for duty by reason of venereal and other forms of disease have been returned to Australia, and a considerable number sent to Malta.

There have been returned to Australia by the *Kyarra* on February 2, the *Moloia* on March 15, the *Suevic* on April 28, and the *Ceramic* on May 4, a total of 337 soldiers who were medically unfit for various reasons, and 341 suffering from venereal disease, or 678 in all. In addition about 450 were sent to Malta. If these soldiers had been added to the list of those reported sick and unfit for duty daily, the number would have considerably exceeded 2,000. The estimate of 2,000 sick and unfit for duty daily was studiously moderate, as pointed out in a private letter to Colonel Fetherston at the time when precise figures could not be immediately obtained.

It is gratifying to find that the amount of sickness is diminishing and that the amount of venereal disease, so far as can be ascertained, is also decreasing.

Strenuous efforts have been made by the A.M.C. to attack both forms of inefficiency by dealing with the causes, and with a view to avoiding future troubles the D.M.S. Egypt has appointed a committee of medical officers to inquire into the causations of the outbreak. It is unlikely that the committee can be very active just at present, because of the prior claims on the time of all concerned owing to the influx of wounded. At a later period it is hoped that an exhaustive report will be furnished for the benefit of future undertakings.

Most strenuous efforts have been made to limit the amount of venereal disease. General Birdwood, Commander-in-Chief of the New Zealand and Australian Army Corps, has personally interested himself in this question, and has through the O.C. First Australian General Hospital arranged for me to visit each troopship on arrival, all leave being stopped from the transport until I have been on board. The practice followed is to interview the commanding officer and the officers of the transports, to explain to them the gravity of the position, and to ask each and all of them to use all the influence he possesses with his men to deter them from exposing themselves to the risk of contagion, to draw their attention to the fact that on the physical fitness of the individual man depends the possibilities of success to the army, and to ask for the loyal and enthusiastic co-operation of every officer in work of such importance from a military point of view, and the point of view of subsequent civil life.

The officers immediately parade the men, address them, and convey to each of them a printed message from General Birdwood. General Birdwood's letter to General Bridges, written during the early part of the stay of the army in Egypt, is handed to the commanding officer to be read by him and his staff. There is no doubt that this systematic procedure has drawn attention to the gravity of the problem. It has always been responded to loyally by the officers concerned, and it has certainly limited the action of young and inexperienced men on their first landing in an Eastern country.

Other steps were taken by Surgeon-General Williams, who on arrival in Egypt called a conference of senior medical officers to consider the gravity of the venereal diseases problem.

It is satisfactory to find, notwithstanding the amount of disease which has existed, and which, while not excessive, is still heavy, that the mortality has not been as serious as it might have been. The mortality in No. 1 Australian General Hospital for February and March was seventeen cases out of a total of 3,150 admitted" (Report ends).

The following return shows the total number of casualties in the Australian Force up to July 16, 1915:

Casualty	Officers	Other Ranks	Total
Killed	110	1,598	1,708
Died of Wounds	46	740	786
Wounded	341	8,404	8,745
Died of Disease	—	43	43
Totals	513	11,555	12,068

The next table shows the average length of stay in hospital of venereal cases at a particular date:

FIRST AUSTRALIAN GENERAL HOSPITAL

Total venereal cases admitted	1,288
Average stay of patients	16 days

THE ENLISTMENT OF THE UNFIT AND ITS CONSEQUENCES

Prior to the arrival of the wounded the medical service was inconvenienced by another circumstance. Men were continually arriving with hernia, varix, and other ailments which they had suffered from before enlistment, and which had been overlooked during the preliminary examination in Australia. In one case a soldier suffering from aortic aneurism arrived in Egypt, and similar instances might be given. The examination of recruits in Australia had been conducted by practitioners in country towns and elsewhere, often under conditions highly unfair to the practitioner. There is no doubt that the government would have been well advised to have withdrawn a few men from private practice altogether, paid them adequate salaries, and made them permanent examiners of recruits.

Experience of war demonstrates most completely the folly of sending any one to the front who is not physically fit. It is apt to be forgotten that in warfare there can be no holidays, or days off, and that the human being must be at his maximum of physical efficiency, and his digestion of the best. If his soundness is doubtful it is better to keep him for base duty at home, on guard duty at the base, or as an orderly in the hospital. It is simply a waste of money, and tends to the disorganisation of the service, to send such people anywhere near the fighting line. We made an attempt at one stage to roughly calculate what the Australian Government had lost in money by the looseness of official examination. It was impossible to make an accurate estimate, but the sum was great.

OPHTHALMIC AND AURAL WORK

When one of us joined the hospital as oculist and aurist and registrar (Lieut.-Col. Barrett) he was informed that specialists were not required, but apparently those responsible had formed no conception of the excessive demands which would be made on the ophthalmic and aural departments. The first patient admitted to No. 1 General Hospital was an eye case, and an enormous clinic rapidly made its appearance. It was conducted somewhat differently from an ordinary ophthalmic and aural clinic, in that (by reason of the remoteness of their camps) some patients were admitted for ailments which would have been treated in the outpatient department of a civil hospital. There were usually from 60 to 100 inpatients and there was an out-patient clinic which rose sometimes to nearly 100 a day. It should be remembered that these included few, if any, serious chronic cases, which were at once referred back to Australia. The amount of oph-thalmic and aural disease was very great. The figures subjoined show the extent of the work done.

From the opening of the hospital to September 30, 1915, the patients treated in the Ophthalmic and Aural Department numbered as follows:

Ophthalmic cases	1,142
Aural, nasal, and throat cases	1,474

There were 246 operations

The ophthalmic cases may be roughly classified as follows:

Ophthalmia (chiefly Koch-Weeks and a percentage		546
Affection of lids		15
Pterygium		8
Corneal opacities		6
Trachoma		17
Iritis		12
Cataract		8
Foreign bodies in the eye		14
Old Injuries		9
Detachment of retina		2
Strabismus		16
Concussion blindness		4
Refraction cases:		
(a) Hypertropia	210	
(b) Myopia	30	
(c) Hypertropic astigmatism	230	
(d) Myopic astigmatism	15 —	485
		———
		1,142
		———

Aural, Nasal, and Throat Cases	
Acute catarrh (middle ear)	95
Chronic " "	315
Cerumen	190

Dry catarrh (Eustachian)	120
Oto-sclerosis	138
Concussion deafness	139
Nasal catarrh	114
Septal deflection	96
Adenoids	74
Polypi	4
Enlarged tonsils	12
Antra and Sinuses	14
Pharyngeal catarrh	11
Aphonia	8
Laryngeal growth	1
	1,474

Operations Performed
Opthalmic

Excision	36
Iridectomy and extraction	11
Removal F. B.	7
Ptertgium	4
Minor operations	6
	64

Aural

Mastoid operations	17
Removal F.B.	3
	20

Nasal

Adenoids	73
Spurs	34
Polypi	14
Tonsils	41
	162

Total performed, 246

The distribution of disease is unusual. In the course of a long and extensive practice one of us (Lieut.-Col. Barrett) had not seen as many cases of adenoids in adults as he examined in Egypt in three months. It seemed that the irritation of the sand containing organic matter caused inflammation and irritation of the naso-pharynx. Of ophthalmia there was a great deal. It was usually of the Koch-Weeks variety, and gave way readily to treatment. There were a few cases of gonorrhœal ophthalmia, two of which arrived from abroad, and all of which did well. After the arrival of the wounded, however, a new set of problems made their appearance. A limited number of men were totally blind, mostly from bomb explosions, and a large number of others had received wounds in one eye or in the orbit.

It soon became evident that an eye punctured by a fragment of a projectile is almost invariably lost. The metal is non-magnetic. It is usually situated deep in the vitreous; it is practically impossible to remove it even if the eye were not infected and degenerate. A still more remarkable phenomenon, however, made its appearance. If a projectile enters the head in the vicinity of the eye, and does not actually touch it, in most cases the eye is destroyed. Whether from the velocity or the rotation of the projectile, the bruising disorganises the coats of the eye and renders it sightless. In all such cases, if the projectile was lodged in the orbit, the eye was removed together with the projectile. The total number of excisions was thirty-six. In no case did a sympathetic ophthalmitis make its appearance. The eyes were not removed unless the projection of light was manifestly defective. A fuller account of the precise ophthalmic conditions will be published elsewhere.

If the general physical examination of recruits was defective, it is difficult to find suitable terms to describe the examination of their vision. Instances were not infrequent where men with glass eyes made their appearance, and there were several recruits who practically possessed only one eye. Spectacle-fitting was the chief work, as many of the recruits required glasses, mostly for near work, but sometimes for the distance. Ultimately the War Office decided to provide the spectacles. In such a war, it is impossible to exclude recruits for fine visual defects, still, men with only one eye can hardly be sent to the front.

One remarkable instance occurred. A man suffering from detachment of the retina had but one effective eye. I gave directions that he should not be sent to the front, but he eluded authority, and reached Gallipoli, where he was hit in the blind eye with a projectile. I subsequently removed the eye.

The work was excessive, but only one life was lost, though on occasion the condition of some of the sufferers was grave to a degree. One of the most remarkable cases of injury was that of a man who was struck below the left eye by a bullet which emerged through the back of his neck, to the side of the median line. The bullet in emerging tore away a large quantity of the substance of the neck, leaving a hole in which a fair-sized wine glass could have been placed. He was a cheerful man, and sat up in bed propped with pillows, because of the weakness of his neck, and observed to a visitor "Ain't I had luck!" He made an excellent recovery.

It is remarkable that there should have been so much refraction work, and there is no doubt that a working optician, *i.e.* spectacle maker, should accompany every army. Men are often just as dependent for their efficiency on glasses as on artificial teeth, and in a war of this character cannot be rejected.

The acute inflammations of the middle ear were of the most severe type, caused temperatures rising to 103° F. and sometimes left men on convalescence as weak as after a serious general illness. The attacks were so vicious that the pathologist, Captain Watson, sought for special organisms, but found only *staphylococcus*. Probably the same group of organisms which caused vicious pulmonary attacks also caused these severe aural inflammations.

Before our arrival in Egypt malingerers in the force who, having enjoyed a holiday trip to Egypt, wanted to go home again, suddenly discovered that they were blind or deaf. For a time the department was fairly busy detecting the wiles of these men. When they discovered, however, that they would be subjected to expert examination, sight and hearing soon returned. A number of devices were resorted to in order to detect the fraud—*i.e.* the use of faradisation, blind-folding, and the like—and it was rarely that the impostor escaped.

OTHER DISEASES: MEASLES AND ITS COMPLICATIONS;
FOOD INFECTIONS

The danger run by an army from measles is very great indeed, and at an early stage the position was surveyed, and an attempt made to limit the trouble. A cable message was sent to Australia, asking that precautions should be taken against shipping measles cases or contacts. At Suez arrangements were made with the Government Infectious Diseases Hospital to admit any patients suffering from measles or infectious diseases who might land with the recruits. In such cases the

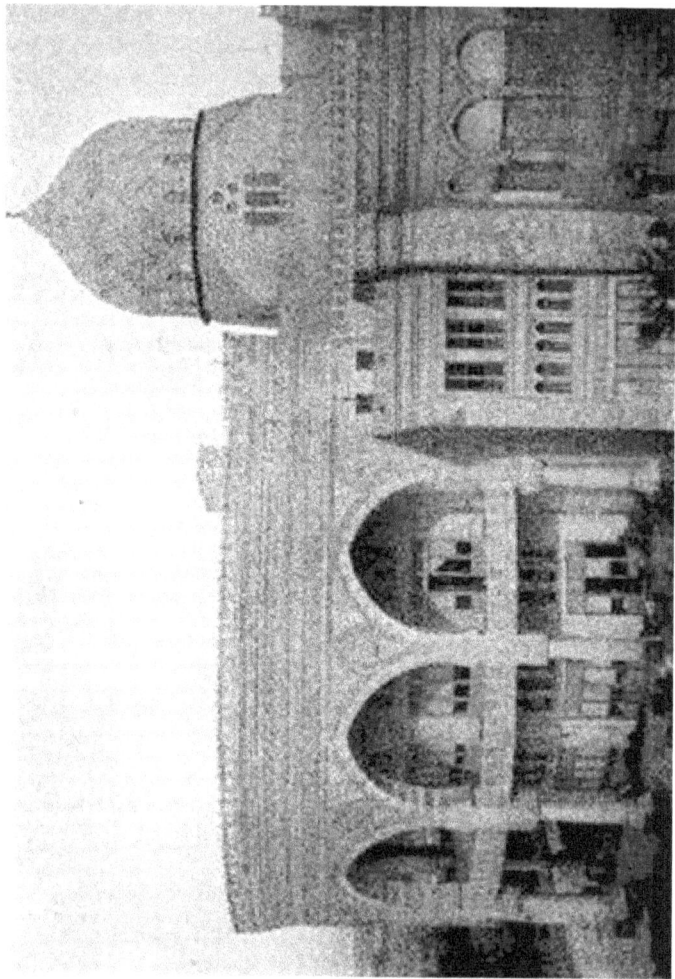

HELIOPOLIS PALACE HOTEL: ROTUNDA AND PIAZZAS.

clothing of the remaining recruits was disinfected before they were allowed to proceed to Cairo. In this way disease was kept out of Egypt as much as possible. In the case of measles it is not simply temporary disablement, but also the complications and *sequelæ* which are to be feared. The experience gained has made us converts to the open-air method of treating such cases, at all events in a rainless country like Egypt. Treated on *piazzas* and in open spaces the cases seem to do better than in hospital wards, and, as far as one can judge without a critical examination, with a lower mortality.

The extent to which the troops suffered from measles and other diseases was the cause of the appointment of a committee to inquire into causation. The committee made some inquiries, but owing to a set of complications never completed its work. There seemed, however, to be a consensus of opinion that the use of the bell tent was objectionable, as it did not ventilate readily, and that the habits of the men contributed to these diseases.

The men were apt to visit Cairo, spend the evenings in the *cafés* or theatres, ride home in the cold nights in a motor car or tram, get to bed at the last moment possible, and then turn out again for a hard day's work. The opinion of the physicians was that the drilling of men suffering from even a moderate cold was a source of considerable danger.

If to these causes be added the neglect of the teeth on the part of many of the men, some explanation may be found for the presence of these diseases. Every effort was made to instruct the men through the regimental officers, and there is no doubt that as time went on the quantity of this type of disease somewhat diminished.

Sunstroke was practically unknown. A number of cases occurred during a severe *khamsin*, but the use of a looser and lighter uniform, and the adoption of sensible hours of work, prevented any recurrence. Of two deaths known to have taken place the cause was only partly due to heat. The men were warned against the risk of *bilharzia*, and as they were provided with shower baths there was no inducement to bathe in the muddy pools and canals where *bilharzia* lurks.

With the provision of dentists another risk was removed, at all events in parts. In hospitals, tooth brushes were supplied in thousands, and every effort was made to get the men to use them.

As the summer wore on, however, another type of disease made its appearance—the intestinal infections which, at first unknown, became so frequent in Gallipoli as to be more serious than fighting. In Gallipoli itself it is difficult to see how they could be prevented. In a limited space there were many dead bodies scantily buried, and consequently myriads of flies. The plentiful use of disinfectant, had it been obtainable, might have been useful, but the difficulties were great. Once the dysenteric organisms were introduced, it was practically impossible to stop the spread of disease.

THE FLY PEST

At the Island of Lemnos, however, which was not under fire, and where there was room, the conditions appear to have been nearly as bad, and it is somewhat difficult to know why the fly pest could not have been got under at Mudros. At Heliopolis at an early stage the fly problem was seriously tackled. A sanitary officer was appointed, and charged with the duty of dealing with this important matter. The following precautions were adopted. All refuse and soiled dressings were placed in covered bins, which were provided in quantity. These were removed once daily. Any moist ground in the vicinity of these bins was watered with sulphate of iron solution, and sprinkled with chloride of lime. Fly papers in great numbers were distributed throughout the wards.

The food in the kitchens, whether cooked or uncooked, was kept under gauze covers or in gauze cupboards. By these means the fly pest was reduced to small proportions. But with the least slackness in administration the flies were again in evidence. It was most instructive to see a floor covered with flies if fluid containing food material had been spilled, and to see dirty clothing covered with masses of flies. A piece of soiled clothing half buried in the desert appears to act as an excellent breeding-place.

It was impracticable in Egypt to cover all the windows and doors with fly-proof netting. The exclusion of the air in the hot weather would have been troublesome, and the best type of netting was not obtainable. Furthermore the precautions already enumerated kept the pest under in Heliopolis.

The fly problem was one of the most serious the army had to face. The passage of a dysenteric stool by a man who is really ill was often followed by the entry into his anus of flies before an attendant had time to intervene. Each of these flies might then become a source of infection and had only to light on a piece of food, cooked or uncooked, to cause further damage.

CIRCULAR ISSUED BY THE OFFICER COMMANDING THE HOSPITAL
Destruction and Prevention of Flies

Outside.

1. No rubbish heaps will be allowed.
2. All manure heaps shall be sprayed twice a week with sulphate of iron—2 lb. to 1 gallon of water.
3. All food in the Arab quarters shall be kept in a closed cupboard.
4. All rubbish boxes and open receptacles shall be removed from the premises and neighbourhood.
5. No receptacles other than iron tins with lids kept closed will be allowed to be used for refuse.
6. Every place on which garbage has been exposed shall be freely sprinkled with chloriated lime.

Wards.

1. All food and receptacles for food shall be kept constantly covered.
2. All spit-cups shall be kept covered.
3. All remains of food shall be removed at once to receptacles which are to be kept covered completely and constantly except when uncovered necessarily to receive waste materials.
4. Sisters-in-Charge shall use a liberal quantity of fly papers. Surgical soiled dressings shall be placed in special bins which shall be kept covered.

Kitchen and Mess Rooms.

1. All food shall be kept locked up or completely covered.
2. All remains of food shall be treated as in the wards. The responsible officer shall use a liberal supply of flat or hanging fly papers.

It need hardly be said that the enforcement of even these simple precautions is more difficult than giving the order.

A good sanitary officer, however, acting on these directions, can and did reduce the fly danger to small proportions. The flies were never exterminated, but were kept well under. The least slackness, however, ended in their rapid reappearance. As they are in all probability the principal cause of the gastro-intestinal infections, the matter is one of the first importance.

Typhoid fever made its appearance, and a proper statistical investigation should be made later on to show the extent of the damage done. The general impression respecting the result of the inoculation to which all the troops were subjected was that the disease was not so frequent and certainly not nearly so fatal as it otherwise would have been. Deaths were few.

The men had not been inoculated against paratyphoid, so that exact conclusions will be difficult to draw even when figures become available.

Many people suffered from Egyptian stomach ache, a form of disease which is as unpleasant as it is exhausting. It manifests itself by repeated attacks of colicky pain, apparently usually associated with the colon. The severity of the pains is remarkable, and the persistent recurrence speedily ends in a considerable degree of exhaustion. It is almost certainly due to food infection.

It is obvious that the business of a sanitary medical officer is not merely to inspect buildings and kitchens, but to spend an hour or two a day in the kitchen quietly watching the preparation of the food and giving the necessary instruction and supervision to those who are preparing it. The inefficiency caused by food infections has probably done more harm than many battles. In the camps similar troubles occurred. By reason of the lack of cold storage and the high temperature, rotten food was not uncommon, and caused outbreaks of incapacitating diarrhoea and *ptomaine* poisoning.

When, however, the problem is surveyed dispassionately, the remarkable feature of the work at Heliopolis and in Cairo was the low mortality, as the following table will show:

BURIALS IN OLD CEMETERY, CAIRO

From Arrival of Australians in Egypt, December 5, 1914, to August 14, 1915

British Imperial Force	77
Australian Imperial Force	155
New Zealand Force	50

In view of this extraordinarily low mortality, it is interesting to comment on human intellectual frailty. It was said that the hospitals were septic, that operations of election could not be performed with safety, that the climate was particularly dangerous, and so forth. One letter which reached us made reference to hundreds of deaths of brave fellows due to faulty camp and hospital conditions. Yet here is the fact recorded that the total deaths in Cairo amongst Australians from disease and wounds to August 14 were only 155. All men tend to generalise on insufficient instances, and the tendency in this case was aggravated by some physical discomfort experienced by the generalisers throughout an unusually warm summer—a discomfort accentuated by overwork and a conscientious devotion to duty under trying conditions.

THE EGYPTIAN CLIMATE AGAIN

Dealing with the surgical side of the matter, nothing was commoner at one time than to hear the statement made that owing to the hot weather septic infections were common, that wounds did not heal as they should in Egypt, and that it was not a suitable place to which wounded men should be sent. While quite agreeing with the critics that a cool climate is always preferable to a hot one, it may be remarked that in the first place summer in Egypt, apart from the *khamsin*, is not excessively hot. The *khamsin* blows for a certain number of days in April, May, and the first half of June. The temperature may rise to 112° or more. The wind blows with a fiery blast, and there is no doubt it is exceedingly trying. But if buildings are shut up early in the morning and opened at night, even the *khamsin* may be made tolerable. After the middle of June, however, there is very little wind. One day is very like another. The midday temperature is from 90° to 95° Dry Bulb, and the nights perhaps 65° to 70° Dry Bulb. The Wet Bulb temperatures are set out in the table previously referred to.

For the most part men slept in nothing but pyjamas. No sheet is wanted until towards the end of August. Whilst it is not pleasant to wake in the mornings in a lather, nevertheless, if a practical and cold-blooded examination be made of the facts, the result shows nothing but discomfort.

Grave septic diseases did not occur. The hospitals were perfectly clean, and at Luna Park in particular we have the testimony of Colonel Ryan that the wounds healed by first intention and that the cases did excellently.

As the garrison of Egypt was a very large one, and as Australian troops were continually pouring into it, it was impracticable even if it had been necessary to take the patients anywhere else. The islands of Lemnos and Imbros were far less suitable even for those who had been injured at Gallipoli, and apart from the inconvenience caused by the heat there was no reasonable ground for complaint in Egypt.

Furthermore the heat is not tropical. It is subtropical, as the Wet Bulb temperatures indicate.

In the First Australian General Hospital every care was taken to minimise the inconvenience; a very large number of excellent ice chests were purchased, an enormous quantity of ice was used, and the necessary steps thus taken to diminish the amount of food decomposition and prevent ptomaine poisoning. Fans and *punkahs* were used, and the nights were quite tolerable.

MEDICAL ORGANISATION IN EGYPT

When the Australian forces pass three miles from Australian shores they cease, at all events technically, to be under Australian control, and pass under the control of the commander-in-chief. On arrival in Egypt they passed under the control of General Sir John Maxwell, G.O.C.-in-Chief, Egypt. The medical section passed under the command of the Director of Medical Services, Surgeon-General Ford. The D.M.S. Australian Imperial Force, Surgeon-General Williams, arrived in Egypt in February and was placed on the staff of General Ford to assist in managing these units. He left for London on duty on April 25, and one of us (J.W. B.) was appointed A.D.M.S. for the Australian Force in Egypt on the staff of General Ford. Later, Colonel Manifold, I.M.S., was appointed D.D.M.S. for Australian and other medical units. Thus the Australian medical units were under the same command as New Zealand or British units, but with separate intermediaries.

THE RISK OF CHOLERA

In view of the risk of cholera, the following note by Dr. Armand Ruffer, C.M.G., President of the Sanitary, Maritime and Quarantine Council of Egypt, Alexandria, was issued and, later on, inoculation was practised on an extensive scale.

DR. RUFFER'S VIEWS ON CHOLERA

(Report begins)
The first point is that although, in many epidemics, cholera has been a water-borne disease, yet a severe epidemic may occur without any general infection of the water supply. This was clearly the case in the last epidemic in Alexandria. Attention to the water supply, therefore, may not altogether prevent an epidemic. The second point is that the *vibrio* of cholera may be present in a virulent condition in people showing no, or very slight symptoms of cholera, *e.g.* people with slight diarrhoea, etc.

The segregation of actual cases of cholera, therefore, is not likely to be followed by any degree of success, because this measure would not touch carriers or mild cases, unless orders were given to consider as contacts all foreign foes, and all soldiers who have been in contact with them. This is clearly impossible.

There cannot be any reasonable doubt, therefore, that if the Turkish army becomes infected with cholera, the British Army will undoubtedly become infected also.

Undoubtedly inoculation is the cheapest and quickest way of protection of the troops, provided this process confers immunity against cholera.

It is very difficult to estimate accurately the protection given by inoculation against cholera. My impression from reading the literature on the subject is that: (1) The inoculations must be done at least twice. (2) The inoculations, if properly made, are harmless as a rule. (3) The inoculations confer a certain protection against cholera. I may add that I arrived at this opinion before the war, when the French editors, Messrs. Masson & Co., asked me to write the article "Cholera" for the French standard textbook on pathology. My opinion was therefore quite unprejudiced by the present circumstances.

The cholera inoculations were harmless *as a rule*; that is, *they were not always harmless*. Savas has described certain cases of *fulminating cholera* amongst people inoculated *during the progress of an epidemic*. In my opinion, the people so affected were in the period of incubation when they were inoculated, and the operation gave an extra stimulus, so to speak, to the dormant *vibrio*. One knows that, experimentally, a small dose of toxin, given immediately after or before the inoculation of the microorganism producing the toxin, renders this microorganism more virulent.

The conclusion to be drawn is that inoculations should be carried out before cholera breaks out.

I am afraid I know of no certain facts to guide me in estimating the length of the period of immunity produced by inoculations. Judging by analogy, I should say that it is certainly not less than six months, that it, almost certainly, lasts for one year, and very probably lasts far longer.

I understand that 90,000 doses of cholera vaccine have been sent from London. I take it that the inoculation material has been standardised and its effects investigated, but, in any case, I consider that a few *very carefully performed* experiments should be undertaken at once in Egypt, in order to make sure of the exact method of administration to be adopted under present conditions.

Probably, a good deal may be done by the timely exhibition of drugs, such as phenacetin, etc., to mitigate the more or less unpleasant effects of preventive inoculation.

As I am on this subject, may I point out the necessity of establishing at the front a laboratory for the early diagnosis of cholera and of dysentery. Cholera has appeared in the last three wars in which Turkey has been engaged, and therefore the chances of the peninsula of Gallipoli becoming infected are great. The early diagnosis of cases of cholera, especially when slight, is extremely difficult and often can be settled by bacteriological examination only.

There never has been a war without dysentery, and almost surely our troops will be infected in time, if they are not already infected. But whereas in previous wars the treatment of dysentery was not specific, the physician is *now* in possession of rapid methods of treatment, provided he can tell what kind of dysentery (bacillary or amoebic or mixed) he is dealing with.

This differential diagnosis is a hopeless task unless controlled at every step by microscopical and bacteriological examination.

The French are keenly aware of this fact, so much so that they have sent, for that very purpose, three skilled bacteriologists, two of whom are former assistants at the Pasteur Institute, to the Gallipoli Peninsula.

(Report ends).

OTHER INFECTIOUS DISEASES

The Infectious Diseases Hospitals were filled mostly with cases of measles and its complications, including severe otitis media. Cases of erysipelas, scarlatina, scabies, and diphtheria were met with in small numbers. In the autumn there was a severe epidemic of mumps.

Through the summer and autumn many cases of diarrhoea and of both amoebic and bacillary dysentery made their appearance. There is good ground for believing that many so-called diarrhoeal cases were dysenteric.

There is little doubt short of absolute scientific proof that the greater part of the intestinal diseases are fly borne.

The following table shows the admissions into the hospital, the deaths, and causes of death, to July 31, 1915.

A subsequent table shows the deaths and causes of death in No. 2 Australian General Hospital from May 3 to August 18.

ADMISSIONS AND DEATHS INTO NO. 1 AUSTRALIAN
GENERAL HOSPITAL

From February to July inclusive

	Admissions.	Deaths.	Cause of Death.
February	1,360	1	Malignant purpura
March	1,791	12	6 Pneumonic group 3 Measles, etc. 1 Meningitis 1 Abscess, liver 1 Tumour, brain
April	1,343	12	2 Pneumonic group 7 Measles, etc. 1 Meningitis 1 Septicæmia 1 Injury
May	2,650	35	27 Wounds (1 tetanus) 1 Meningitis 1 Poliomyelitis 1 Cardiac 1 Pancreatitis 1 Appendicitis 3 Pneumonic group
June	2,862	20	11 Wounds 1 Perinepritis 1 Nephritis, chronic 1 Septicæmia 1 Broncho-pneumonia endo- carditis 1 Pneumonia 1 Meningitis 2 Enteric 1 Dysentery
July	2,099	19	6 Wounds 1 Fracture, tibia 1 Enteric 6 Dysentery 1 Diphtheria 3 Meningitis 1 Enteritis

In May and June 5,512 men were admitted, of whom 1,219 were Australians and New Zealanders in camp, 2,967 Australians and New Zealanders from the Mediterranean Expeditionary Force, 1,050 British, and 276 Naval Division from the same force.

AUSTRALIAN IMPERIAL FORCE

Return showing Number of Deaths at No. 2 Australian General Hospital, Ghezireh From May 3, 1915, to August 18, 1915

Australian M.E.F

Sickness	2
Wounds in Action	9

British M.E.F.

Sickness	nil
Wounds in Action	1

R.N.D. M.E.F.

Sickness	1
Wounds in Action	nil

New Zealand M.E.F.

Sickness	1
Wounds in Action	nil

Australian Force in Egypt

Sickness	1

D. MacKenzie, Captain
Secretary and Registrar, No. 2
General Hospital

Ghezireh
August 18, 1915.

This chapter would be incomplete unless proper acknowledgment were made of the most valuable post mortem demonstrations given by Major Watson.

CHAPTER 8

Venereal Diseases

The venereal-disease problem has given a great deal of trouble in Egypt as elsewhere. The problem in Egypt does not differ materially from the problem anywhere else, but a number of fine soldiers have been disabled more or less permanently.

When the First Australian Division landed in Egypt and camped at Mena, the novelty of the surroundings and the lack of intuitive discipline resulted in somewhat of an outbreak, both with regard to conduct and to sexual matters. Both of these phases have been greatly exaggerated, but nevertheless there was substantial ground for apprehension, and the following letter from General Birdwood, Commander-in-Chief of the Australian Army Corps, to the officers commanding units was sufficient evidence of the necessity for action.

For Private Circulation only

Divisional Headquarters, Mena,
December 18, 1914.

The following letter written by Major-General W. R. Birdwood, C.B., C.S.I., C.I.E., D.S.O., Commanding the Australian and New Zealand Army Corps, to Major-General W.T. Bridges, C.M.G., Commanding the First Australian Division, has been printed for private circulation.

V. C. M. Sellheim,
Colonel, A.A. and Q.M.G.

Headquarters: Australian and New Zealand Army Corps,
Shepheard's Hotel, Cairo,
December 27, 1914.

My Dear General,

You will, I know, not misunderstand me if I write to you about the behaviour of a very small proportion of our contingents in Cairo, as I know well that not only you, but all your officers and non-commissioned officers and nearly all the men must be of one mind in wishing only for the good name of our contingents.

Sir John Maxwell had to write recently complaining of the drunkenness of some of our men in the Cairo streets. During Christmas time some small licence might perhaps have been anticipated, but that time is now over, and I still hear of many cases of drunkenness, and this the men must stop.

I advisedly say 'the men must stop,' because I feel it is up to the men themselves to put a stop to it by their own good feeling. I wonder if they fully realise that only a few days' sailing from us our fellow-countrymen are fighting for their lives, and fighting as we have never had to do before, simply because they know the very existence of their country is at stake as the result of their efforts.

We have been given some breathing time here by Lord Kitchener for one object, and one object only—to do our best to fit ourselves to join in the struggle to the best advantage of our country. I honestly do not think that *all* of our men realise that this is the case. Cairo is full of temptations, and a few of the men seem to think they have come here for a huge picnic; they have money and wish to get rid of it. The worst of it is that Cairo is full of some, probably, of the most unscrupulous people in the world, who are only too anxious to do all they can to entice our boys into the worst of places, and possibly drug them there, only to turn them out again in a short time to bring disgrace on the rest of us.

Surely the good feeling of the men as a whole must be sufficient to stop this when they realise it. The breathing time we have left us is but a short one and we want every single minute of it to try and make ourselves efficient. We have to remember too that our Governments of the Commonwealth and Dominion have sent us here at a great sacrifice to themselves, and they fully rely on us upholding their good name, and indeed doing much more than that, for I know they look to us to prove that these two contingents contain the finest troops in the British Empire (whose deeds are going down in history), whom they look forward to welcome with all honours when we have done our share, and I hope even more than our share, in ensuring victory over a people who would take all we hold dear from us if we do not crush them now.

But there is no possibility whatever of our doing ourselves full justice unless we are every one of us absolutely physically fit, and this no man can possibly be if he allows his body to become sodden with drink or rotten from women, and unless he is doing his best to keep himself efficient he is swindling the government which has sent him to represent it and fight for it. From perhaps a selfish point of view, too, but in the interests of our children and children's children, it is as necessary to keep a 'clean Australia' as a 'White Australia.'

A very few men can take away our good name. Will you appeal to all to realise what is before us, and from now onwards to keep before them one thought and only one thought until this war is finished with honour—that is, a fixed determination to think of nothing and to work for nothing but their individual efficiency to meet the enemy.

If the men themselves will let any who do not stick to this know what curs they think them in shirking the work for which it has been their privilege to be selected, then, I know well, any backslidings will stop at once—not from thoughts of punishments, but from good feeling, which is what we want.

I have just been writing to Lord Kitchener telling him how intensely proud and well-nigh overwhelmed I feel at finding myself in command of such a magnificent body of men as we have here; no man could feel otherwise. He will, I know, follow every movement of ours with unfailing interest, and surely we will never risk disappointing him by allowing a few of our men to give us a bad name. This applies equally to every one of us, from general down to the last-joined drummer.

Will you and your men see to it?

Yours very sincerely,

W. R. Birdwood.

Those who possessed any experience of life could not but realise that 18,000 particularly vigorous fine men, brought up in a country where discipline is conspicuous by its absence, and landed for the first time in a semi-eastern city such as Cairo, were likely to behave in such a manner that a small minority would get into trouble. Active steps were taken to meet the difficulties, and to prevent recurrence of the outbreaks when the Second Division and other reinforcements arrived.

General Birdwood accordingly issued the following circular:

WARNING TO SOLDIERS RESPECTING VENEREAL DISEASE

Venereal diseases are very prevalent in Egypt. They are already responsible for a material lessening of the efficiency of the Australasian Imperial Forces, since those who are severely infected are no longer fit to serve. A considerable number of soldiers so infected are now being returned to Australia invalided, and in disgrace. One death from syphilis has already occurred.

Intercourse with public women is almost certain to be followed by disaster. The soldier is therefore asked to consider the matter from several points of view. In the first place if he is infected he will not be efficient and he may be discharged. But the evil does not cease even with the termination of his military career, for he is liable to infect his future wife and children.

Soldiers are also urged to abstain from the consumption of any native alcoholic beverage offered to them for sale.

These beverages are nearly always adulterated, and it is said that the mixture offered for sale is often composed of pure alcohol and other ingredients, including urine, and certainly produces serious consequences to those who consume it. As these drinks are drugged, a very small amount is sufficient to make a man absolutely irresponsible for his actions.

The General Commanding the Australasian Forces, therefore, asks each soldier to realise that on him rests the reputation of the Australasian Force, and he is urged at all costs and hazards to avoid the risk of contracting venereal disease or disgracing himself by drink.

This leaflet was entrusted to Lieut.-Col. Barrett to deliver to troops on arrival, and he accordingly visited Port Said and Suez, interviewed the officers on the transports, and fully explained the position to them. They were requested to use their influence with the men in the direction of restraint. Subsequently after the destruction of the *Konigsberg* the transports began to arrive at irregular intervals and it became impossible to meet the officers at the ports. They were then interviewed at Abbassia or Heliopolis, and later still by order of General Spens, G.O.C. Training Depot, the men themselves were addressed on the day of their arrival. The form of address was simple. The dangers of infection were pointed out to them—particularly as regards typhoid fever, dysentery, *bilharzia*, and venereal disease. They were shown how the first three diseases could be avoided.

So far as venereal disease was concerned they were informed that the matter was in their own hands. They were asked to imitate the Japanese, and by their own efforts preserve their health with the same care that they bestowed on their rifles or their ammunition, the preservation of health and arms being equally important. Passages from the famous rescript of the Emperor of Japan before the Russian war were quoted in which it was stated in substance that if the normal proportion of sick existed in the Japanese army defeat was a practical certainty; but that if they followed the direction of their medical officers and took the same care of their bodies as they took of their equipment, the number of troops saved thereby would make all the difference in the ensuing conflict.

General Birdwood asked for the whole-hearted and enthusiastic co-operation of all officers in doing their best to control their men, and to prevent them from exposing themselves to the risk of venereal disease. Some little time before the issue of the circular 3 *per cent.* of the force were affected by venereal disease on any one day. Fortunately, as a result of the efforts made, the tendency was to diminution, but the amount of venereal disease was still sufficiently great to give concern and anxiety.

There is no doubt that the action of General Birdwood prevented outbreaks and limited the amount of disease. It is also equally true that in spite of his efforts the amount of disease was too large to be contemplated with equanimity.

The Venereal Diseases Hospital, Abbassia, was nearly always full, but from time to time drafts of men were sent back to Australia. One draft of 450 soldiers was sent to Malta early in the campaign. The principle involved in the policy of returning them to Australia was as follows. In Egypt they were useless as soldiers, whether suffering from gonorrhœa or syphilis. They required a large number of medical men and attendants to take care of them. They knew they had disgraced themselves and were a source of trouble to everyone concerned. On shipboard they could not get into trouble. They were more likely to be cured, and could then be returned to Egypt, and if not cured could be treated in Australia at leisure.

Against this policy the argument was used that diseases were being

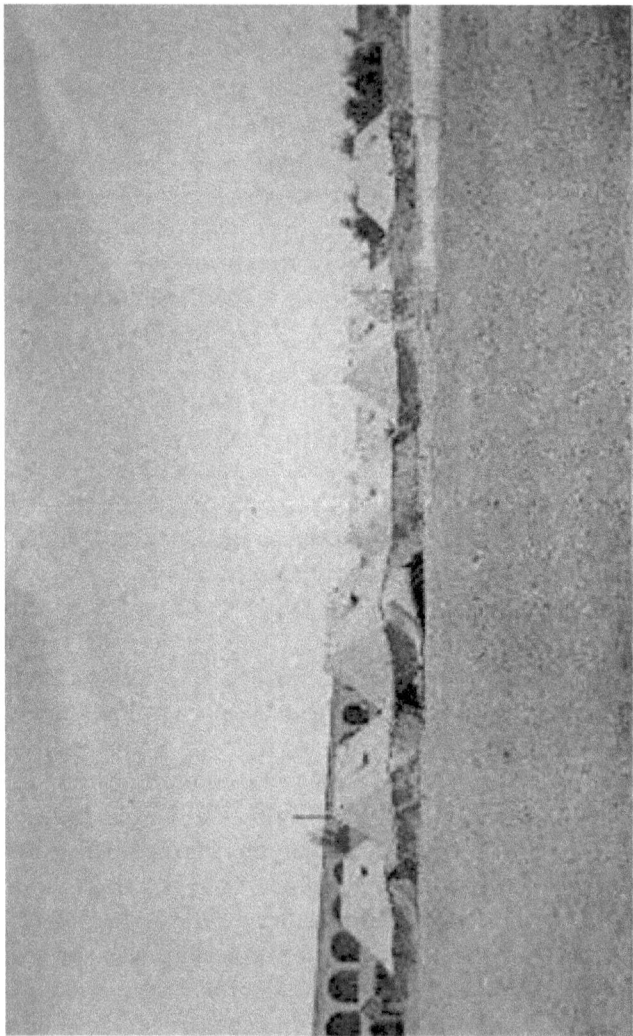

VENEREAL DISEASES HOSPITAL, ABBASSIA.

introduced into Australia, but as a matter of fact a minority of the men suffering from venereal disease brought it from Australia to Egypt. They arrived at Suez suffering from gonorrhœa contracted in some cases at Fremantle. Furthermore the business of those conducting the campaign was to wage a successful war, and to keep the base as free from encumbrance as possible. The total number returned to Australia in this way was as follows:

From February to September 14, 1,344, and in addition 450 were sent to Malta.

At first they were sent in ships with other cases and sometimes segregated on board, but difficulties arose at the Australian ports. The people who welcomed the returned soldiers were sometimes enthusiastic in greeting venereal cases by mistake, and sometimes non-venereal cases were regarded with suspicion because they came from a ship known to convey venereal patients. It was finally decided by the Australian Government that venereal cases should be conveyed in ships by themselves, the first consignment of 369 being sent in the *Port Lincoln*.

A certain number of the gonorrhœal cases recovered and became fit for service, but too often they relapsed.

The authorities were fully alive to the damage which was being done, and persistent and earnest attempts were made to deal with it from many different points of view. General Maxwell issued an order prohibiting the sale of drink after an early hour (10 p.m.) in the evening, and also prohibiting soldiers from being found in Cairo after an early hour. There is no doubt that both of these directions proved to be of considerable value.

MORAL CONDITIONS IN CAIRO

Something must be said, however, about the moral conditions in Cairo, about which exaggerated and perverse notions seem to be entertained. Cairo, like all large cities in the world, possesses its quota of prostitutes, who differ only from prostitutes elsewhere in that the quarters are dirtier and that the women are practically of all nationalities, except English. The quarter in which they live is evil-smelling, and is provided with narrow streets and objectionable places of entertainment. It contains a considerable infusion of Eastern musicians and the like, and is plentifully supplied with pimps of the worst class. These men were promptly dealt with by the police, the authorities giving the most sympathetic assistance to the military.

As in other countries, there were graduations in the class of women employed, and the personal impression gained by the authorities was that the danger of infection was greatest from those at the top and the bottom of the social scale. Prostitutes who were registered were examined by a New Zealand gynecologist, who did the work very thoroughly, and conscientiously, and with kindness. Women who were free from disease were furnished with a ticket indicating that they were healthy. At the beginning of the war there were 800 of these women in Cairo, but as the war progressed the number grew to 1,600. The arrangement then differed in no way from the arrangements in Melbourne or Sydney except that the surveillance of the police was direct, and medical examination was insisted upon. It further had this advantage over those of Melbourne and Sydney, that the women were confined to one particular part of the city, and no one need come in contact with them unless they wanted to. Consequently for those who went to this quarter there is no excuse, since they acted deliberately.

Prophylaxis

At the same time, when all these measures were weighed in the balance—plain speaking to the men on arrival, police surveillance, medical examination, etc.—it was felt that more might be done. A number of medical officers accordingly gave instruction to their men in the means of effecting prophylaxis and of preventing infection in the event of association with these women. The medical officers acted entirely on their own responsibility. They advised the men to avoid the risk, but as they knew a certain number would not take their advice in any circumstances—in fact the men said as much—they showed them how to avoid infection if they would take the necessary trouble.

Result of Prophylaxis

In the case of our own unit, the First Australian General Hospital, trouble was taken to explain in detail the consequences of venereal diseases to the men, and to those with whom they would be associated in later life. They were asked to refrain from taking the risk, but for those who would not take the advice—and there was bound to be a percentage—the necessary directions and material were provided for preventing infection. The result was challenged by a medical officer, and an immediate examination of all the men made, when it was found that in the whole of the unit only one man was infected. In other words, the precautions taken had practically stamped the disease out of the unit, and shortly after arrival in Cairo.

Once the disease was acquired the treatment was troublesome to a degree. The men knew they were disgraced; they would probably be sent back to Australia; and in some cases, those of the finer men, the consequences were serious. Mostly, however, they developed an attitude of sullenness and indifference, a tendency to lack of discipline, and they rendered the management of camps difficult. These troubles to a large extent disappeared when a suitable hospital was established.

Soldiers' Clubs

But another and constructive side of the matter appealed forcibly to those concerned. Why not supply for the benefit of the men places of entertainment with music, refreshments, and the like, similar to and better than those which the prostitutes supplied, but minus the prostitute. In other words, why not give a healthy and reasonable alternative? After consultation with His Excellency Sir Henry MacMahon, with the G.O.C.-in-Chief, General Sir John Maxwell, and with the D.M.S. Egypt, General Ford, the Australian Red Cross Society determined to combine with the Y.M.C.A. and establish clubs for the soldiers in central positions where these requirements would be met. They accordingly established a club at the quay in Alexandria, and a magnificent open-air club in the Esbekieh Gardens, Cairo. They were both immediately successful, and have played a most important part in the further limitation of the amount of venereal disease. It is difficult to give statistical evidence, but there is no doubt that by these various means a sensible difference has been produced in the incidence of disease amongst the troops.

The Duty of the Medical Officer

We have never wavered from the conviction that any one suffering from venereal disease should be treated by a medical practitioner exactly like any other sick person. In military service, however, an added element makes its appearance in that the soldier by his act has rendered himself unfit, and consequently must suffer some pains and penalties. It is no answer to say that other men have exposed themselves and have not become infected. The fact remains that he has by a deliberate and avoidable act deprived his country of the value of his services. And whilst the doctrine of punishment should not be pushed too far, he certainly should not receive the same general treatment as other soldiers, and the policy of his prompt return to Australia and deprivation of pay was in the circumstances the best one.

In the Venereal Diseases Hospital, Abbassia, the men were well treated. They were well fed, and a certain amount of Red Cross help was given to them.

Many proposals were made which were not carried into effect: for example, placing of the prostitute quarter "out of bounds" and the posting of sentries. It was realised that the immediate effect of this action would have been to drive women to the vicinity of the camps, and that it was impracticable. Another practicable proposal was made, which, however, was not carried into effect—the creation of dispensaries in the vicinity of the prostitute quarter, so that immediate treatment could be obtained. In many camps such dispensaries were established by the medical officers.

The essence of the problem was learnt by a brigadier-general who visited a number of young educated men in one of the camps, and asked them for their viewpoint on the subject. Their answer was that which every medical officer knows full well: that many men were influenced by the appeals which had been made to them, but that a percentage have indulged in this way throughout their adult life, and intend to continue to do so irrespective of anything medical officers, chaplains, or generals may say to them. It is this fundamental position which every reformer must face. So long as a sufficient number of men determine to adopt this policy, and so long as there is a sufficient number of women prepared to cater for them, the problem of venereal disease will continue to be acute in every country.

The opinion has been expressed elsewhere that the world will not be rendered more or less moral by the abolition of venereal disease, and instruction in the mode of preventing infection should be an essential part of education. Because people are immoral there is no reason why they should acquire gonorrhœa or syphilis. If the *lex talionis* is to be enforced, the logical way to deal with the matter is to refuse treatment to all the infected, and to let them die or become disabled. But the most thorough-going Puritan shrinks from adopting so terrible a policy. One method or the other, however, must be adopted—there can be no half-way house. And if the decision be in favour of eradicating the disease, it is essential to firmly face and grapple with the problem.

Wassermann Tests

The examination of the cases showed that gonorrhœa was far

more common than syphilis, and a series of Wassermann determinations showed that the cases of soft sores did not give a syphilitic reaction in the early stages. Captain Watson of the First General Hospital made a number of determinations in order to try to settle this important point.

THE POLICY TO BE ADOPTED

In spite of all that was done, 1,344 men were returned to Australia disabled, and 450 were sent to Malta. If a calculation be made of the cost of sending these men to Egypt and back, and of their pay before they were infected, some idea may be formed of the enormous sum of money the Australian Commonwealth wasted on men who were a drag and hindrance to the army machine.

The government should, on the raising and equipping of a volunteer army, treat it as older countries treat a standing army by issuing instructions to the men.

When the hospitals left Australia neither officers nor men received instructions, and not until the arrival of Surgeon-General Williams in Egypt was any serious collective action taken. He at once called a conference of medical officers and did what he could to limit the extent of disease.

The governmental action—or lack of action—is unsound, since the man who contracts disease is severely punished, but adequate attempts are not made to prevent him acquiring it. The notable departure made in the case of Cairo was the effort to make the men understand clearly what these diseases meant to them as soldiers and as citizens; to remove temptation from them as far as possible, and with the aid of the Australian Red Cross to give them a reasonable, healthy, and decent alternative. Nothing the Australian Red Cross has done (or is likely to do) is more important than the establishment of the Soldiers' Clubs. Nothing has been more successful or is likely so to redound to the credit of that great institution. And yet, under the new Constitution of the Australian Red Cross, not a shilling can be devoted in the future to such purposes.

VENEREAL DISEASES CONFERENCE

The following are brief notes of a conference of senior medical officers convened by Surgeon-General Williams.

Reference was made to the gravity of the problem with which the force was faced. It was estimated that about 1,000 men of the First and

Second Australian Divisions are suffering from venereal disease on any one day, and of these a large number are incapacitated from work. The proportions seemed to be much greater than those of other forces, such as the Territorials, in Egypt. The displacement of so large a proportion of men and the ultimate consequence of numerous infections, rendered it necessary to take a comprehensive view of the position, and to endeavour to take some action to minimise the damage done. It was proposed to ask each officer present to furnish the secretary with a general statement of the number of cases treated under their command, specifying them under three headings—syphilis, soft chancre, and gonorrhœa. The information so obtained would form the basis of a report to headquarters. The problem was considered under five headings:

1. Military assistance.

2. Use of prophylaxis.

3. Treatment—general and special.

4. Establishment of convalescent depots—accommodation and position.

5. Ultimate destination of affected men.

1. *In what way can the military authorities give assistance?*—There are three ways in which they can approach the problem:

(*a*) They may decide that all areas known to contain brothels are out of bounds.

(*b*) They can provide adequate military control by military police organised under a competent officer, with one or more junior medical officers to assist him.

(*c*) That punishment can be inflicted on those men who break bounds and expose themselves to the risk of venereal infection. It might be desirable to reduce the pay of men found in those areas whether suffering from venereal disease or not.

2. *Prophylaxis.*—Officers were invited to discuss the question whether it would not be advisable to establish prophylactic depots in various parts of Cairo. Men to report immediately after exposing themselves to infection, and by cleanliness and the use of medicaments prevent infection. Circulars couched in plain and sensible language might be issued to the troops, conveying to them a knowledge of the risk they run, and the fact that if infected they will take back to Australia a disease which would reduce their value as citizens.

3. *General and Special Treatment.*—Suggestions from officers present were invited.

4. *Convalescent Depots.*—Was it right that the hospital should be crowded out with venereal cases, which demanded very much time and attention from the staffs? If the hospital was placed near the scene of military action the wounded might suffer from the amount of attention required for venereal cases. Most venereal cases required rest in the main, and this could be obtained in convalescent depots.

5. *The ultimate destination of the affected men.*—Two courses are open: The men may be treated in Egypt, or sent back to Australia.

(*a*) If they are kept in Egypt and the Australian Expeditionary Force is moved to the front its medical services would be depleted, and medical men of great ability and experience would be left behind to take charge of venereal cases when their services were required at the front.

(*b*) If on the other hand the Australian and Imperial Government could utilise some ships for the accommodation of these men, those who were cured could be sent to the front, and those who could not be cured could be sent back to Australia at once. But such ships would require special staffing so that the existing units should not be depleted in order to provide staffs.

In the discussion which ensued it was represented that there was a difficulty in placing areas out of bounds, as the brothels would be moved to other areas. Prophylaxis was regarded as most important. Isolation tents could be set apart in the regimental lines where men could be treated on return from leave. Cases of syphilis should be sent to Australia.

The reduction of pay is forbidden by King's Regulations, and although the Minister for Defence in the Commonwealth of Australia authorised such reduction, it is only for such period as the troops are in Egypt.

It was agreed that cases of syphilis should be returned to Australia, as there is no chance in Egypt of treating them efficiently, and even if such treatment were available the men would not be fit for duty for from four to six months.

It was pointed out that at least 100 men left Australia with the First Division suffering from venereal disease.

The chief difficulty seemed to be what venereal cases would ultimately be of service to a fighting line, and to properly arrange for

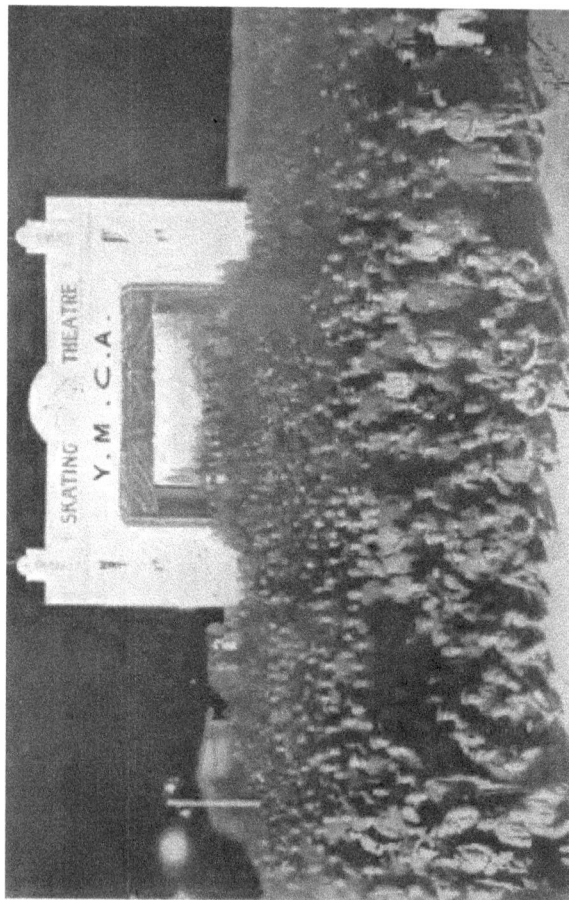

Soldiers' Club, Esbekieh, Cairo.

them during convalescence; in other words, when and how men considered unfit for further service should be returned to Australia. Officers were asked to recollect that the future of these soldiers was to be considered and the part they would play in civil life. In the American Navy unbounded shore leave had been given, and had some effect in checking the disease. In the British Navy it was an offence not to report "exposure."

The Soldiers' Clubs are fully described in the chapter on the Red Cross. They were rendered possible by an alliance between the Y.M.C.A. and the Australian Branch British Red Cross. To the Y.M.C.A., who managed them, the best thanks of Australia should be given, for Australians will never fully know what they owe to Mr. Jessop and his assistants. Unfortunately, the Australian Branch British Red Cross subsequently decided that help should be given *only* to sick and wounded. Although convalescents frequent these clubs, the view was taken—we think wrongly—that Red Cross funds could not be used for their support. We feel sure that when Australians fully understand the matter the decision will be reversed.

CHAPTER 9

The Red Cross Work: Its Value and Limitations

The British Red Cross Society, Australian Branch, was founded by Her Excellency Lady Helen Munro Ferguson, wife of the Governor-General of Australia, on the outbreak of war. On previous occasions unsuccessful attempts had been made to found an Australian Red Cross Society. On this occasion the movement was most successful, although many people then (like some people now) were quite unable to understand the distinction between the Red Cross movement and military administration.

The Red Cross Society in Australia undertook the collection of funds for immediate transmission to the British Red Cross Society for prompt use in the field. Branches were formed in each State and committees were formed by the wives of the various governors. Thus a rough-and-ready arrangement was made prior to the adoption of a constitution. It was considered far more important to do the work than to waste time holding meetings and devising a constitution. Those who could not afford to give money were invited to make clothing or to contribute articles of various kinds.

Specifications of the clothing requisite were given, and patterns furnished so that it might be readily made on approved design. It is not too much to say that the majority of the inhabitants of the Continent were soon engaged in some way or other in helping the Red Cross movement. The ball-rooms of the respective Government Houses were used as depots.

The depot at Federal Government House, Melbourne, was an excellent model. People were invited to send their donations irrespective of their number or their kind. These were received and receipted, and were then sorted into bundles of similar articles by lady volunteers. They were then placed in cases by volunteer packers, mostly experienced men from various warehouses, and were finally dispatched to Europe as opportunity offered.

The arrangement of these details fell largely on the Council and Secretary of the Branch (one of us, J. W. B.) in Australia acting under the direction of the President, Her Excellency Lady Helen Munro Ferguson. Very great difficulty was experienced in finding space in merchant ships for the conveyance of the goods. Space was found on the transports, but there was not the same security for delivery. In addition the hospitals of the transports were provided with such equipment as the officers commanding desired.

When, however, the Lines of Communication Units were ordered to Egypt, another problem arose, and the Australian Red Cross Society decided to properly equip these units both with money and goods. For this purpose £10,000 was set aside and forwarded to London. It was handed to the British Red Cross Society and kept available for the officers commanding the five hospitals, the requisite sum of money to be allotted to them by Surgeon-General Williams, C.B., the Director of Medical Services in Australia, who had proceeded to Europe. At the time it was supposed that these five hospitals were proceeding to France.

In addition large quantities of goods were available at the British Red Cross Society in London, and large quantities of goods were given to the several hospitals for dispatch with their equipment. When, however, the hospitals were sent to Egypt a new situation arose. There were many other medical units in Egypt besides the hospitals. There were the Field Ambulances and the Regimental Medical Officers, and Surgeon-General Williams regarded them as equally worthy of assistance.

On his arrival in Egypt at first, in December, and subsequently in the middle of February, the scope of the British Red Cross, Australian Branch, in relation to Australian troops had extended far beyond the original intention. The action taken is described in the following report sent to the President and members of the Council, British Red Cross Society, Australian Branch, on my resignation (Lieut.-Col. Barrett) from that body on September 9, 1915. I did not at any time receive any instructions from Australia, and acted in the manner which seemed best after consultation with local authorities.

Report on the Work of the Australian Branch British Red Cross in Egypt, from March to September 3, 1915

By James W. Barrett, *Lieut.-Colonel, Lately Executive Officer, Australian Branch British Red Cross Society*

Report presented to the President and Members of the Council of the Australian Branch British Red Cross Society

The First Australian General Hospital arrived in Egypt in January 1915. I was associated with it as Registrar and Oculist and had nothing to do with the Red Cross movement beyond assuming responsibility for any Red Cross goods which belonged to the Hospital.

When leaving Melbourne Colonel Ramsay Smith was informed that there would be room for 100 tons of Red Cross goods in the *Kyarra*. When, however, the *Kyarra* reached Melbourne her holds were full and no Red Cross goods were taken on board. There were consequently not any Red Cross goods available at No. 1 Australian General Hospital for some considerable time after arrival in Egypt.

Surgeon-General Williams, C.B., arrived in Egypt in the middle of February, and at once proceeded to organise the Red Cross movement. He had been entrusted with £10,000 which was to be expended by the officers commanding medical units according to the plan set out later. He at once took action, and money was distributed to a number of hospitals and medical units. This distribution was of the utmost service.

When Red Cross goods began to arrive in Egypt he sought a suitable store. Finding nothing in Cairo at a reasonable price, he established a store in the basement of the Heliopolis Palace Hotel, No. 1 Australian General Hospital, for which, of course, no rental was charged. The store was placed under the immediate charge of the Orderly Medical Officer, Captain Max Yuille, and under my general direction. The distribution of money and collection of goods from ships was effected by General Williams through his own office in Cairo.

General Williams left for London on duty on April 25, leaving me in charge of the Red Cross work, and leaving his Warrant Officer, Mr. Drummond, in his office to continue the collection of goods and the clerical work.

Soon after he had left, the crisis of May and June took place. Wounded and sick were poured into Cairo on a scale probably never known or equalled before. There have been occasions on which a much larger number of men have been wounded, but probably never

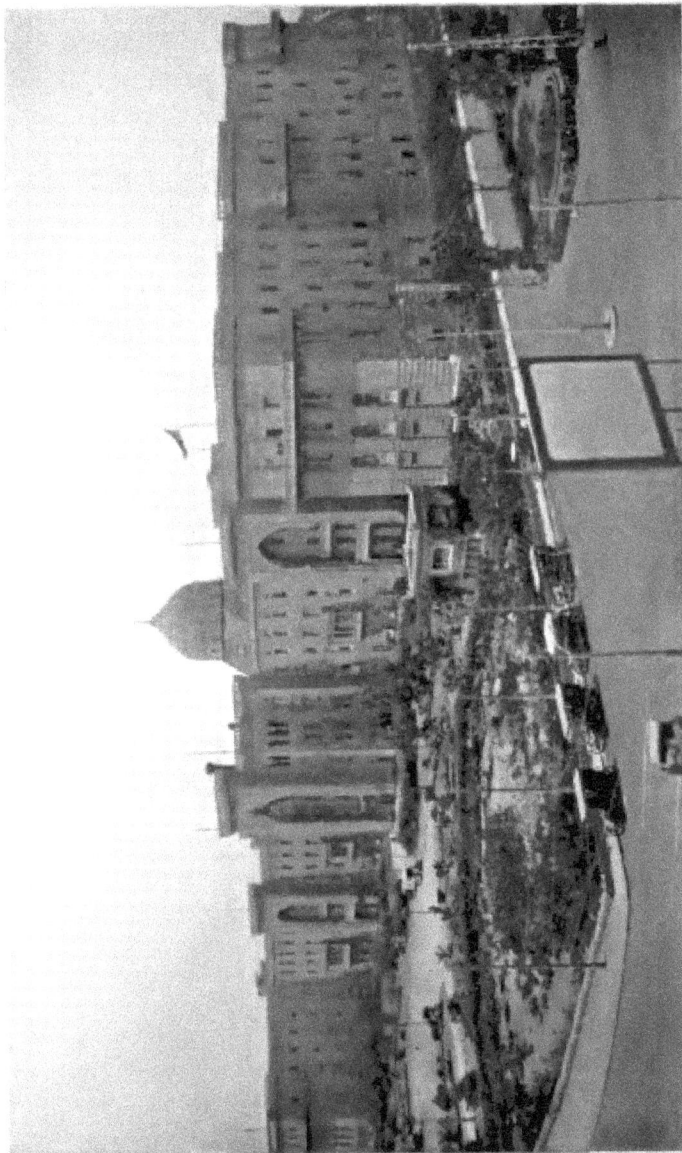

Heliopolis Palace Hotel.

any occasion in history in which so many wounded men have been handled in so limited a space. Fortunately preparation had been made by the D.M.S. Egypt, Surgeon-General Ford, D.S.O., and the D.M.S. A.I.F., Surgeon-General Williams, C.B., who instructed the O.C. First Australian General Hospital, Colonel Ramsay Smith, and myself as registrar to take over extra buildings and provide equipment. It was this action which prevented a disaster, and whilst not strictly a Red Cross matter was greatly aided by Red Cross equipment.

During this crisis I was instructed by the D.M.S. Egypt, Surgeon-General Ford, and the O.C. Australian Intermediate Base, Colonel Sellheim, to visit various hospitals in Egypt—both in Alexandria and the provinces—to interview the Australian wounded and supply all reasonable comforts. In accordance with this order, money and goods, either or both, were sent to various hospitals as set out in the various tables.

It so happened that the British Red Cross Society possessed neither money nor goods at the inception of the crisis, and the authorities were profoundly grateful for the help which the Australian Branch afforded. The British Red Cross, Egyptian Branch, at a later stage received large supplies of money and goods which were freely distributed. The fact that goods could be obtained from the British Red Cross Society, Australian Branch, soon became known, and many requisitions were received. The list of goods available was widely circulated and in no instance was the requisition of any officer commanding not complied with. It was always completed to the extent of our resources. Periodical reports of the work done were prepared and forwarded to the President of the Australian Branch British Red Cross Society, Melbourne.

Whilst the work was at its height a message from Australia reached His Excellency Sir Henry MacMahon, in consequence of which two committees were formed on June 3, 1915—a General Egyptian Committee and an Executive Committee.

The members were:

General Committee:
    President, His Excellency Sir Henry MacMahon
    Lord Edward Cecil
    Sir Alexander Baird
Executive Committee:
    Sir John Rogers

Dr. Ruffer
Surgeon-General Williams.
Lieut.-Colonel Barrett.

Sir Courtauld Thomson is the Commissioner in the Mediterranean for the British Red Cross Society, and Sir John Rogers and Dr. Ruffer Deputy Commissioners in Egypt.

Surgeon-General Williams and Lieut.-Col. Barrett were appointed members of the Executive Committee of the British Red Cross Society in Egypt.

There was no amalgamation of the two branches, but by this arrangement each was kept informed of the activity of the other and wasteful overlapping was avoided.

Members of the General Committee investigated the work of the Australian Branch, were consulted in matters of policy, and received and investigated any complaints. They were most helpful.

General Williams returned to Egypt on June 21, made a tour of inspection, and visited the Australian wounded. He reported to the government, and finally left for London on duty on June 29. On this occasion he took with him his office staff, and consequently the administration fell largely into my hands.

On July 13, however, I learned by cable from Australia that two commissioners had been appointed in terms which seemed to place them in entire control of the Red Cross movement.

As it was desirable that other medical officers should be associated with the movement. Colonel Ryan, Colonel Martin, and Lieut.-Col. Springthorpe were invited by His Excellency Sir Henry MacMahon to join the Executive Committee.

Mr. Adrian Knox, K. C., the first of the commissioners, arrived in Cairo on August 11, and the second commissioner, Mr. Brookes, reported on August 27. I endeavoured to help them in every way that was possible, and finally asked to be relieved of the work on September 9, expressing my willingness, however, to continue to aid in any way they desired. My relationship to them has been cordial, and I am very glad if I have been able to be of any assistance.

I now propose to deal with the operations of the society under various headings:

1. *Finance.*—The original fund in the hands of Surgeon-General Williams was operated upon by him in London, in Malta, and in Egypt. It was only in Egypt that I was concerned with it, and to a lim-

ited extent. It was most helpful, and great service was rendered during the crisis by the prompt distribution of money.

When the General Committee, of which His Excellency Sir Henry MacMahon is President, was formed, separate funds were forwarded to him in response to a cable from me indicating that more money was wanted. I suggested the supply of another £10,000, but when, on July 9, £18,000 had been received it became obvious that operations were contemplated on a more extensive scale than had hitherto been thought necessary. I have prepared a summary of the amounts distributed to medical units from both funds, and given an account of the method adopted.

The Red Cross Society originally intended that £10,000 was to be expended by the officers commanding medical units, and General Williams embodied the direction in the following circular, to which I subsequently added a memorandum in further explanation of new conditions which had arisen.

Australian Imperial Force

Received from Surgeon-General W. D. C. Williams, Director Medical Service, A.I.F., the sum of . . . . .stg. to be utilised and accounted for by me in terms of Circular Letter No. E 1/15, dated 13-2-15.

. . . . .O.C.

Place . . . .

Date. . . . .

Australian Imperial Force

Circular Letter No. E 1/15.

O.C.,

1. Forwarded herewith the sum of . . . .
. . . . .stg. to be expended by your authority and direction on such articles as you may consider requisite for the general improvement of equipment, stores, or other items which in your opinion will conduce to the general well-being and comfort of the patients in hospital under your command.

2. Attached receipt forms to be signed in duplicate and returned to me.

3. When three-fourths of the amount allocated to you has been expended, you will furnish this office with expenditure vouchers in duplicate. This will enable me to keep the High Commis-

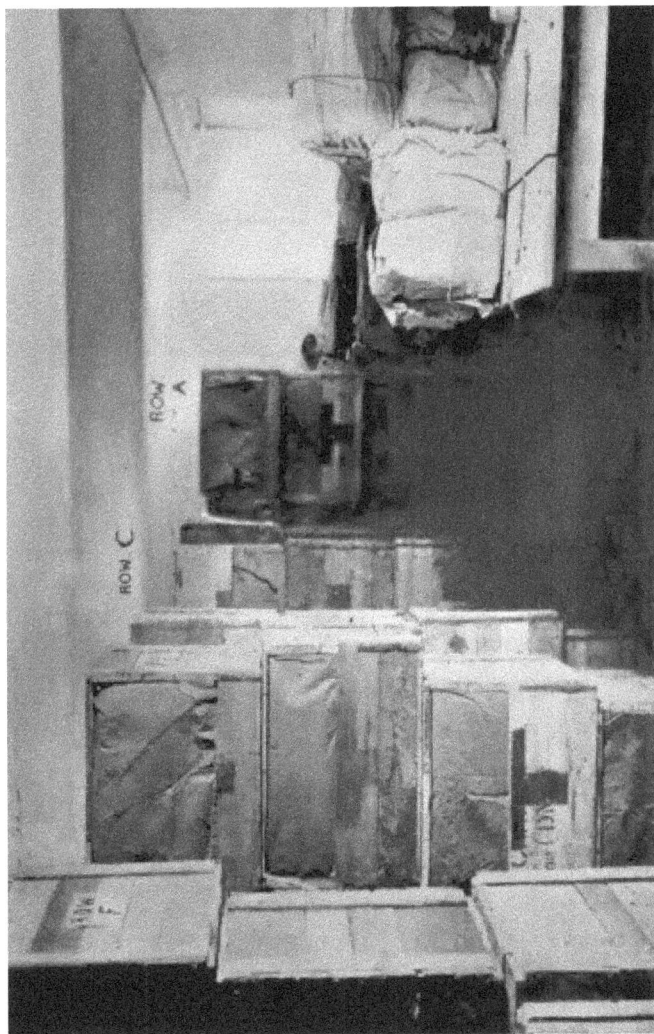

INTERIOR OF RED CROSS STORE: UTILISATION OF CASES FOR SHELVING.

sioner informed as to how the moneys are being spent, and to arrange for further grants if considered necessary.

Surgeon-General,
Director Medical Services, A.I.F.

(*Copy*)

May 20, 1915.

O.C.

Govt. Hospt.

Tanta, Damanhour and Shebin el Kom.

1. I enclose herewith cheque for (£50/£25/£25) to be expended in terms of the circular letter attached. Will you please sign the accompanying receipt in duplicate and oblige.

2. It is not desired that the expenditure of the money should be restricted to Australians, as such a course would, I think, in a hospital be impracticable and undesirable. If, however, this is used for all the Allied troops under your care, then the next instalment which may become necessary might well be provided from the "Military Hospitals Fund" or the "Egyptian Red Cross Fund."

3. I shall be glad if you will communicate to the men in the hospital the fact that comforts are being supplied from the Fund of the British Red Cross Society (Australian Branch), the administration of which fund is in the hands of Surgeon-General W. D. C. Williams, C.B.

(Signed)

James W. Barrett,
Major,
for W. D. C. Williams,
Surgeon-General.

GRANTS OF MONEY MADE TO VARIOUS HOSPITALS FROM RED CROSS FUNDS

Hospital or Medical Unit, etc.	Amount in Egyptian pounds.
First Australian General Hospital and Auxiliaries	1376,42.5
Second Australian General Hospital .	682,50
Share of Rent of Luna Park for three months	117,00
Y.M.C.A. (including stationery, building fund, Soldiers' Café, and sundry accounts)	982,08.6

Venereal Hospital, Abbassia	. .	48,75
Deaconess Hospital, Alexandria	. .	78,00
European Hospital, Alexandria	. .	48,75
Government Hospital, Tanta	. .	53,62.5
No. 21 General Hospital, Alexandria	.	97,50
Convalescent Home, Al Hayat, Helouan		341,25
Convalescent Home, Ras el Tin, Alexandria	. . . . .	97,50
A.D.M.S., First Australian Division	.	292,50
First Stationary Hospital	. . .	195,00
Second Australian Stationary Hospital	.	196,24.7
First Casualty Clearing Station	. .	146,25
Fourth Field Ambulance	. . .	290,00.2
First Light Horse Field Ambulance	.	97,50
Second Light Horse Field Ambulance	.	195,00
Third Light Horse Field Ambulance	.	48,75
Fifth General Hospital	. . .	97,50
Fifteenth Stationary Hospital	. .	97,50
17th General Hospital	. . .	146,25
Bombay Presidency Hospital	. .	58,50
Government Hospital, Alexandria	.	48,75
Convalescent Camp, Mustapha	. .	48,75
Government Hospital, Damanhour	.	24,37.5
Government Hospital, Shebin el Kom	.	34,12.5
5th Indian General Hospital, Alexandria		48,75
Government Hospital, Benha	. .	5,00
Greek Hospital, Alexandria	. . .	29,25
Government Hospital, Suez	. .	24,37.5
Red Cross Depot, Suez	. .	48,75
Ras el Tin Hospital, Alexandria	.	195,00
15th General Hospital, Alexandria		48.75
		£E.6340,26

The Egyptian pound is to the British pound sterling as 100:97·5.

In addition, a considerable amount of money had been spent in other countries. There was, however, no knowledge in Egypt of the sum which would be ultimately available. Furthermore, in the absence of instructions from Australia, no serious departure had been made from the policy originally laid down. In fact I am doubtful to a degree whether any Red Cross movement should in normal conditions go

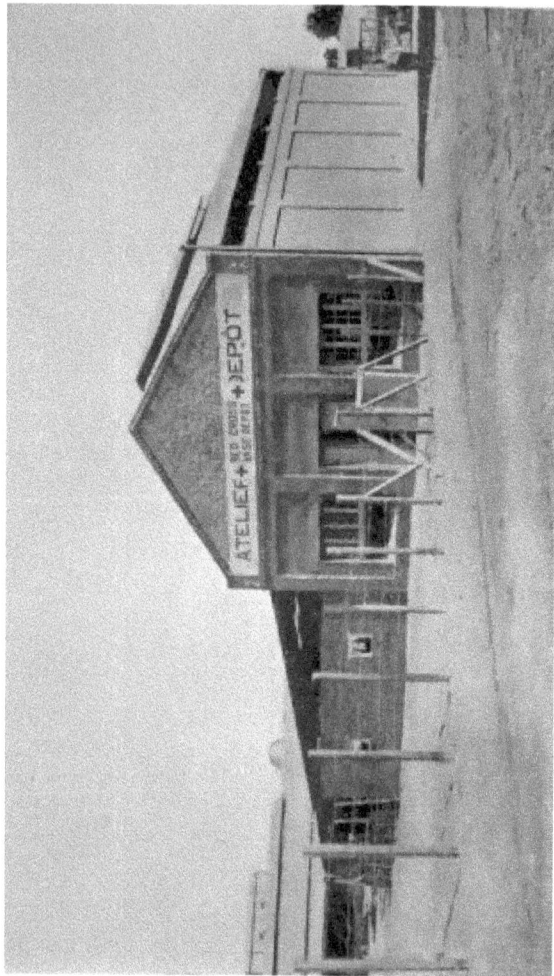

Red Cross Base Depot, Heliopolis.

beyond the successful policy adopted.

2. *Red Cross Store.*—Goods received were passed into the Red Cross store, the contents of the cases ascertained as far as possible, and entered in books kept for that purpose. They were issued on requisition signed by the officer commanding any medical unit. Corresponding entry was made in the book of issue, and the difference between the stock received and that issued from day to day was shown in the form of a stock sheet. Stock-taking was effected from time to time.

The store was staffed at first by two nurses and three orderlies, later it was staffed by a sergeant and six or seven orderlies who were approved by the military authorities. The staff therefore consisted of myself, with my own clerical staff, the orderly officer of the hospital, Captain Max Yuille (latterly Captain Dunn), the sergeant and seven orderlies, together with extra helpers at times. The store was connected by telephone with the hospital, and every effort made, compatible with the excessive demands on the time of all, to manage it in a methodical manner.

3. *Receipt of Goods.*—The receipt of goods has, owing to the peculiarities of Egypt and the circumstances of the war, given a good deal of trouble, and I am making it the subject of a separate memorandum. It may suffice here to say that it will never be satisfactory until the Red Cross Society in Australia cables, when the ship leaves Fremantle, precisely the number of packages on board, the port of destination, and the probable time of arrival of the ship; and also accurately informs the officers commanding the ship of the nature of the Red Cross goods on board.

In this connection it may be interesting to note the following letter from Colonel Onslow, who has just arrived by the *Runic* in Egypt, and who, but for the printed instructions drawn up by me and conveyed to him at Suez, would not have known that any Red Cross goods were on board:

Continental Hotel, Cairo,
September 13, 1915.

Lieut.-Colonel Barrett,
A.A.M.C.

My Dear Sir,
You will remember that on Saturday last you asked me to write to you regarding the Red Cross Stores on the Transport A 54 *Runic* of which I was in military command.

When I took command on August 9 in Sydney I had no information as to there being any Red Cross Stores on board except that one of the ladies of the Red Cross Committee had told me that a few stores were to be put on board and would be at my disposal if needed for the troops under my command.

Subsequently I saw some half a dozen cases which I assumed to be those to which she had alluded.

On arrival at Suez, September 9, the printed instructions as to disposal of Red Cross Stores were handed to me. This caused me to make inquiries. The ship's purser knew nothing of any such stores and they were not shown in the manifest.

But from the chief officer I learned that a large number of which he had an incomplete list had been placed in one of the holds. It was even then too late for me to ascertain their number or nature, as I was in the midst of disembarking returning ship stores, etc. They were therefore landed without the required list.

But if either a wireless had been sent to me a day or two beforehand, or if the persons responsible for shipping had informed me in Sydney, there would have been no difficulty whatever. Under the lack of system which would seem to prevail in shipping these stores from Australia it would not be surprising if they were overcarried and lost.

Yours faithfully,

(Signed)   J. Macarthur Onslow,
                                                              Colonel.

I publish this letter simply to show the difficulties and to indicate the magnitude of the task. I do not think anyone is to blame, but rectification is wanted.

A huge commercial concern has gradually grown up and now requires firm paid commercial management. The Australian Red Cross has become a gigantic Commercial Institution with attendant advantages and disadvantages.

It should be remembered that goods are shipped in Australia from at least six different ports separated by distances of hundreds of miles, that nearly the whole of the work has been amateur, and that it is difficult to inaugurate a proper business system rapidly.

The following are the printed directions referred to by Colonel Onslow:

From A.D.M.S., Australian Force,
Headquarters, Cairo.
To O.C. Troopship ——

1. Will you please instruct a medical officer to make a list in duplicate of the surplus medical stores and Red Cross goods, including ambulances, on the ship. He will hand one list to the representative of Australian Intermediate Base (Captain Clayton) and retain the other.

2. Will you please detail a medical officer, or if that be impossible another commissioned officer, who will see that these goods are put on the train, and travel with them to their point of destination.

3. At the place of destination he will hand them over with an inventory to a representative of A.D.M.S. Australian Force (Lieut.-Colonel Barrett), from whom he will obtain a receipt. He will not, under any circumstances, hand them over to anyone else, or take any verbal receipt.

4. If it be impossible to send the goods by passenger train they may proceed by goods train, in which case an N.C.O. or orderly must be detailed to travel in the brake van; and deliver the goods to a representative of A.D.M.S. Australian Force (Lieut.-Colonel Barrett) in precisely the same way.

5. You will please detail a fatigue party of sufficient strength for unloading the goods from the transport and placing them on the train, and in addition supply any guard that is necessary to protect them until this work is completed.

6. It is undesirable in any circumstances to send goods by troop train. It is much better to send them by goods train.

7. Will you please convey these orders in writing to the medical officer or officer concerned. If any conflicting orders be issued he can then produce this authority.

A.D.M.S. Australian Force.

4. *Distribution of Goods.*—The distribution of goods was effected on requisition signed by the O.C. of the medical unit requiring them, transport was provided by the Red Cross Society to the railway station (usually by motor lorries) and at public expense on the railways. I soon learnt that in Egypt in time of war there is no certainty of the delivery of the goods to the proper quarter unless someone is sent with them. The railway officials will frequently hand over goods to a

military officer without obtaining a receipt. Accordingly one or more orderlies were sent with every train conveying Red Cross goods. They handed the goods to the consignee and brought back the receipt.

In the Australian hospitals the distribution of goods was effected by two methods. Anything wanted from the central store could be obtained by requisition signed by the O.C. of the hospital, and countersigned by myself as Red Cross officer. Very large quantities of goods were thus transferred from the central store to the quartermaster's department. They were then issued in the ordinary way by requisition of the sisters or medical officers, and those receiving them were not aware whether they were receiving Red Cross goods or ordnance goods. The system had the merit of extreme simplicity, and was very speedy in its operation. It certainly seemed at the time far less important that patients should know where the goods came from than that they should obtain them promptly. Later on the expediency of putting a Red Cross label on everything supplied became obvious and was adopted as a policy.

5. *Scope of Operations.*—At first the operations of the Society were confined to Egypt, but soon, in conjunction with the British Red Cross, goods were forwarded to the Dardanelles and elsewhere. The tables show the quantity of goods sent to transports in the Mediterranean and transports leaving for Australia. No request was ever refused. When dispatching goods to the Dardanelles it was considered better to act, as far as possible, through the British Red Cross Society.

On July 5 I wrote to General Birdwood, Commanding Officer A. and N.Z. Army Corps, asking him whether I could establish a Red Cross store at Anzac. He replied that it was impossible, but at his suggestion a Red Cross store at Mudros in the island of Lemnos was organised in conjunction with the British Red Cross Society. The Army Medical Corps at Anzac was then advised to requisition on Mudros. The difficulties, however, of landing goods at Mudros were very great—so great that the British Red Cross Society was compelled to buy launches and lighters. The Australian Red Cross Commissioners are about to supplement the purchase. The tables show the quantity and character of the goods sent forward in spite of many difficulties. It was often necessary to send an orderly in the hospital ship to Mudros and Anzac to ensure delivery.

6. *Other Activities.*—The British Red Cross Australian Branch arranged through the Y.M.C.A. for the free distribution of stationery to

the soldiers in hospitals in Egypt. With the assistance of the Y.M.C.A. and some English ladies in Cairo a number of committees were formed to entertain the sick and wounded in various ways. A cinema was purchased, a small orchestra was engaged to visit the hospitals, bands of ladies agreed to take flowers and the like to the hospitals, and everything was done that could be done to render the tedium of convalescence less objectionable.

Large recreation huts were built at many of the hospitals at the expense of the Australian Branch.

This phase of the work should not be passed over without the most handsome acknowledgment to the English ladies in Cairo. These public-spirited ladies, headed by Mrs. Elgood, thoroughly organised what I may call the lighter side of hospital work, and not only by their personal attention, but also by their tactful skill, succeeded in making the conditions of the sick and wounded much more comfortable. Furthermore although we left Australia knowing that the Y.M.C.A. did good work in camps, yet the practical experience of the Y.M.C.A. work in Egypt has left an indelible impression on our minds. Headed by Mr. Jessop, their secretary, there was no service in connection with the sick and wounded which they failed to render when provided with the proper means. We felt the utmost confidence in entrusting them with any undertaking, provided that the position was clearly defined and provided that they were not hampered in their activities.

In passing it may be said that until June 15 the shortage of nurses and medical officers was considerable. Of lay helpers there were few in Cairo during the summer, and the principle was invariably adopted of using all existing agencies to cover the ground, the necessary support being given by the Red Cross Society. It was on this principle that Mrs. Elgood acted, it was on this principle that the Y.M.C.A. acted, and it is on this principle that all great organisations can be most successfully conducted. If it had become necessary to create an independent organisation to provide cinemas and bands, to disburse stationery in Egypt and at the Dardanelles, distribute flowers, fruit, games, etc., a very large number of soldiers would have been employed who were much better employed otherwise. Furthermore, they would not have done the work as well as Mrs. Elgood's staff or the Y.M.C.A.

7. *Issue of Purchased Goods.*—As the fund grew in volume it was decided to spend some of it in the purchase of articles desired by the men. A vote was taken at No. 1 Auxiliary Convalescent Depot (Luna

Park) to ascertain the articles the men most desired—see appendix. Boxes containing a number of articles were issued to every patient on admission. This has involved an expenditure rising to £500 per month.

A sample box has already been sent to Australia. In each box the following note was placed:

> The object of the Australian Red Cross Society is to provide comfort and help to the wounded and sick soldiers, such as hospital clothing, invalid comforts, tobacco, toilet necessaries, books, magazines, newspapers, and the like, and also recreation huts for entertainment, etc.
>
> These comforts are supplied over and above the hospital necessaries which the Commonwealth of Australia furnishes on so liberal a scale.
>
> The Society hopes that your stay in the hospital will be short and pleasant, and that your convalescence will be rapid so that you can speedily serve your country again. The Society asks you to accept the contents of this box as an indication of Australia's desire to help you.

8. *Convalescent Home at Montazah.*—The Montazah palace, which was owned by the late Khedive, was offered to Lady Graham by H.H. the Sultan as a Convalescent Home for soldiers. The British Red Cross Society and the Australian Branch combined and agreed to find £3,500 to equip it.

This beautiful hospital consists of a number of buildings situated on the shore of the Mediterranean, with artificial harbours and provision for bathing, fishing, and boating. It is now in excellent order and is most successful.

While I think it was right to take a share in the erection of this convalescent home, which indeed could not have been obtained as a military hospital, it immediately raised in mind the consideration of the propriety of the Red Cross conducting hospitals in any circumstances. It is of course the English practice, and the special circumstances of Great Britain may make it necessary to erect Red Cross hospitals. The Commonwealth of Australia has never prevented the establishment of as many hospitals as may be considered necessary in the field.

In my judgment it is better to limit the conduct of military hospitals and convalescent hospitals to official authority, leaving the Red Cross to supplement the work in the way already indicated. Otherwise the Red Cross is simply doing governmental work. The Red Cross may do the work very well indeed, but the advantage is not obvious.

9. *Motor Transport.*—The motor ambulances presented by the Australian Branch have been housed in two garages, one at Heliopolis and the other at Gezira. They were both designed by Surgeon-General Williams and provided from Red Cross Funds. It is not too much to say that the organisation of the motor transport assisted materially in saving the position.

For a long time, with the exception of some New Zealand ambulances, there were no other ambulances in Egypt. At Heliopolis a repairing plant was installed at Red Cross expense in order to reduce the cost of repairs.

There is no doubt that the British Red Cross Australian Branch was at the outset of exceptional service because it possessed on the spot stores, money, and motor transport.

10. *Bureau of Inquiry.*—The British Red Cross Society instituted a bureau of inquiry in order to obtain supplemental information about the sick and wounded. Inquiries on an elaborate scale are made at the office of the Commonwealth Government, but certain supplementary and private inquiries can be made with profit. The British Red Cross Society was requested to undertake such inquiries and to charge Australian Red Cross for the extra assistance necessitated.

11. *Hospital Trains.*—At an early stage steps were taken to equip hospital trains running from Alexandria to Cairo with everything the officers in charge required.

Furthermore, arrangements were made at Red Cross expense to provide a restaurant car on all trains conveying sick and wounded to Suez. Detailed arrangements can be found after the following lists. This arrangement has proved of great benefit. The men obtained free lime juice and water and their rations. They could purchase in addition comforts at bed-rock prices.

The innovation may seem a small one, but it was not effected without considerable trouble owing to shortage of rolling stock.

Prepared by Staff-Sergeant Hudson

Unit.	Articles.	Cases.	Pkgs.
First Australian General Hospital	76,350	462	39
No. 1 Auxiliary Convalescent Depot	3,377	22	
No. 2 Auxiliary Convalescent Depot	11,340	78	7
No. 3 Auxiliary Convalescent Depot	6,393	74	13
Infectious Diseases Hospital, Choubra	6,303	7	
Ras el Tin Convalescent Home	19,562	65	8
Al Hayat Convalescent Home	36,050	92	2
No. 2 Australian General Hospital, Ghezira	25,437	75	4
Mena Australian Hospital	2,705	4	2
Venereal Diseases Hospital, Abbassia	7,626	22	2
Hospital ships and transports	46,350	19	
Imbros Rest Camp Hospital	650	70	
Kasr el Aini	13,372	11	
Greek Hospital, Alexandria	1,381		
Colonel Bryant, Lemnos	23,236	127	8 sacks
4th Field Ambulance, Dardanelles	8,472	2	

1st Stationary Hospital, Lemnos . . .	42,333	107	12 sacks
2nd Stationary Hospital, Lemnos . . .	187	107	13 sacks
7th Field Ambulance, Polygon Camp, Cairo .	4	2	
2nd Light Horse Field Ambulance, Maadi, Cairo	6,056	2	
2nd Light Horse, Lemnos	7,985	2	
Captain Dunlop, 18th Battalion . . .	37		
Captain Williams, Hqrs. 2nd Austr. Division .	30		
No. 4 Auxiliary Convalescent Depot . .	754		
Heliopolis Dairy Company for 1st A.G.H. .	800		
Zeitoun Convalescent Camp	2,250	13	
6th Light Horse . .	560		
Dr. Hastings . . .	500		
No. 17 General Hospital, Alexandria . . .	3,532		
Deaconess Hospital . . Alexandria . . .	1,733	6	
Egyptian Army Hospital, Abbassia . . .	708	6	
2nd Indian General Hospital	6,486		
Dr. Oulton, Tanta Hospital	3,899		
Mustapha Barracks, Alexandria . . .	4,585		

New Zealand Mounted Rifles . . .	736	1	
Lancashire Fusiliers .	1,116		
No. 15 General Hospital, Alexandria . . .	4,199		
Military Hospital, Cairo .	244	1	
School Hospital, Port Said	700		
Red Cross Hospital, Said-eh School . . .	3,456	2	
No. 4 Base, Medical Depot, Alexandria . . .	13,032		
Convalescent Hospital, Ismailia . . .	1,904		
French Convalescent Hospital, Alexandria . .	2,294		
Ordnance Office Base, Alexandria . . .	9,528		
European Hospital, Alexandria . . .	740		
4th Field Ambulance .	1,250		
Total . . .	411,974	1,357	110

LIST OF RED CROSS GOODS SUPPLIED FROM STORE APART FROM OTHER GOODS PURCHASED AND SUPPLIED

Aprons (surgical) . . .	260
Blankets	5,875
Cholera belts . . .	7,400
Hot-water bottles . . .	407
Bandages	51 cases
,, ...	200
Books	87 pkgs.
Caps	2,010
Caps (surgical) . . .	266
Dressing-gowns . . .	184
Handkerchiefs . . .	46,298
Housewives . . .	776

Cardigan jackets.	.	.	.	3,483	
Hospital jackets .	.	.	.	269	
Pneumonia jackets	.	.	.	341	
Old linen .	.	.	.	90	cases
Mufflers	.	.	.	3,662	
Masks (surgical) .	.	.	.	24	
Nightingales	.	.	.	495	
Overalls (surgeons')	.	.	.	243	
Pillows	.	.	.	2,945	
Pillowslips .	.	.	.	24,501	
Pyjamas	.	.	.	17,300	
Pyjama trousers .	.	.	.	881	
Pipes .	.	.	.	1,570	
Quilts	.	.	.	43	
Sheets	.	.	.	7,240	
Draw sheets	.	.	.	4,032	
Shirts (flannel)	.	.	.	24,876	
Shirts (cotton)	.	.	.	9,913	
Hospital shirts	.	.	.	4,725	
Socks	.	.	.	70,725	
Bed socks .	.	.	.	1,018	
Toilet soap.	.	.	.	2,789	cakes
,, ,,	.	.	.	4	cases
Slippers	.	.	.	5,878	
Towels	.	.	.	43,914	
Medical towels	.	.	.	4,183	
Undershirts (flannel)	.	.	.	12,333	
Underpants (flannel)	.	.	.	5,588	
Vaseline	.	.	.	284	
Face washers	.	.	.	37,665	
Binders	.	.	.	200	
Hospital bags	.	.	.	334	
Soldiers' kit bags	.	.	.	4,710	
Air cushions	.	.	.	17	
Tooth brushes	.	.	.	6,885	
Tooth paste	.	.	.	1,552	
Sea kit bags	.	.	.	717	
Hair brushes	.	.	.	1,047	
Hair combs	.	.	.	1,081	
Ointment .	.	.	.	208	

Playing cards	.	.	.	.	723
Pencils	.	.	.	.	176
Safety pins	.	.	.	.	380
Rubber sheets	.	.	.	.	6
Mosquito nets	.	.	.	.	1,251
Insect powder	.	.	.	.	314 pkts.
Sponges	.	.	.	.	2,756
Tobacco	.	.	.	.	2,379 plugs
,,	.	.	.	.	16 cases
Cigarettes	.	.	.	.	3,741 pkts.
,,	.	.	.	.	1 case
Biscuits	.	.	.	.	64 cases
Extract of beef	.	.	.	.	45 ,,
Soap	.	.	.	.	1,120 bars
,,	.	.	.	.	70 cases
Gooseberries	.	.	.	.	66 ,,
Glaxo	.	.	.	.	38 ,,
Milk	.	.	.	.	36 ,,
Beans	.	.	.	.	20 sacks
Peas	.	.	.	.	13 ,,
Jam	.	.	.	.	172 cases
Syrup	.	.	.	.	54 ,,
Tomatoes	.	.	.	.	51 cases
Milk and cocoa	.	.	.	.	5 ,,
,, ,,	.	.	.	.	69 tins
Pineapples	.	.	.	.	98 cases
Apricots	.	.	.	.	49 ,,
Honey	.	.	.	.	8 ,,
Dried apples	.	.	.	.	47 ,,
Dried peaches	.	.	.	.	115 ,,
Pears	.	.	.	.	43 ,,
Foodstuffs	.	.	.	.	77 ,,
,,	.	.	.	.	55 pots
Malted milk	.	.	.	.	6 cases
Chocolate and sweets	.	.	.	.	2 ,,
,, ,,	.	.	.	.	634 ,,
Extract of malt	.	.	.	.	3 ,,
Rolled oats	.	.	.	.	1 case
Lactogen	.	.	.	.	7 cases
Ground sheets	.	.	.	.	22

Cloth caps	2,984
Games	65
Walking-sticks	16 bundles
,, ...	687 loose
Writing-pads	1,206
Envelopes	28,470 pkts.
Lemons	15 cases
Glass towels	325
Sun glasses	108
Hot-water bottle covers . .	260
Dusters	773
Mattresses	9
Swabs	7 cases
,, ...	500
Candles	1 case
Cane chairs	70
Toilet paper	45 cases
Puddings	1 case
Preserved fruit . . .	47 cases
Linen coats	388
Cushions	115
,, ...	3 cases
Fly whisks	725
,, ...	2 cases
Knives	30
Spoons	95
Wine	8 cases
Deck chairs and camp stools .	340
Bales of clothing . . .	25
Brassards	200
Shaving-brushes . . .	1,801
Skin coats	10
Cotton thread . . .	50 reels
Toilet paper	100
Nail brushes	24
Jug covers	100
Mittens	675

	Articles.	Cases.	Sack.
1st Stationary Hospital, Lemnos	42,333	107	12
2nd ,, ,, ,,	187	107	13
Imbros Rest Camp . . .	650	70	
Col. Bryant, for Distribution, Dardanelles	23,236	127	8
2nd Light Horse, Lemnos .	7,985	2	

Agreement made for Provision of Refreshments to Soldiers on Invalid Trains

1. The Restaurant Car can be placed on the train and the cost of same, £7 10s., guaranteed by Lieut. Colonel Barrett.

2. Meals will be provided for Commissioned Officers, P.T. 20 lunch or dinner, P.T. 5 afternoon tea, at stated times.

3. Meals and afternoon tea will be provided for N.C.O.s in the Restaurant Car at half price.

4. Sandwiches, P.T. 1, and non-alcoholic drinks (soda water, lemonade, etc.), P.T. 1, will be served in the cars by the attendants of the Restaurant Car to soldiers who desire to purchase them.

5. In addition, water will be provided in each carriage for the use of soldiers in *fantasses*, and lime juice will be supplied, two bottles in each carriage, free.

Notice to this effect will be posted in every carriage on the troop train.

July 1, 1915.

12. *Soldiers' Clubs.*—Reference has been made in the chapter on Venereal Diseases to the damage done to Australian troops in Egypt by venereal disease. Reference has also been made to the establishment of soldiers' clubs and recreation huts in various places to provide a counter-attraction to those entertainments furnished by the prostitute and her degraded male attendants. After the various repressive steps already referred to had been taken, an earnest attempt was made to organise this constructive work. The valuable assistance of Mr. Jessop and the Y.M.C.A. was again invited. The Y.M.C.A. proposed to build in Alexandria on the sea front a large building to be used as a central soldiers' club, and to be available for convalescents and the healthy. The Y.M.C.A. had only £250 available and required £1,000. The British

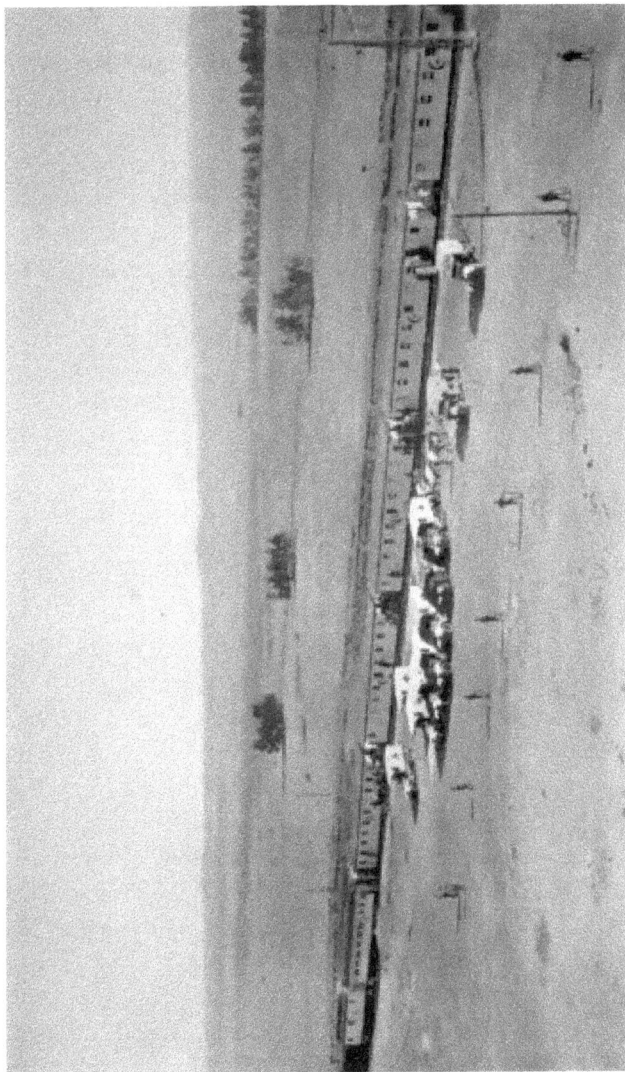

HELIOPOLIS SIDING: ARRIVAL OF WOUNDED.

Red Cross Society was appealed to and hesitated.

A cable was dispatched to London, and an expenditure of £250 authorised. Surgeon-General Williams, after consultation with His Excellency Sir Henry MacMahon, the G.O.C.-in-Chief, Sir John Maxwell, and the D.M.S. Egypt, General Ford, decided to make a grant of £500 in addition for the purpose. The club was opened on September 12, and from its opening was a pronounced success. The soldier on leave, tramping about the streets of Alexandria, gets leg-weary and falls an easy victim to the wiles of the various agents abroad. He now can visit his own club, where the entry is free to all men in uniform. He there receives war telegrams, stationery, cheap and excellent meals, and enjoys various forms of entertainment. He meets his friends, and can spend the time under the most pleasant conditions. The building already requires extension, as the pressure on the accommodation is so great.

Similar action was taken in Cairo, where after many unsuccessful attempts the Rink Theatre in the beautiful Esbekieh gardens was obtained, owing to the sympathetic help given by His Excellency Sir Henry MacMahon and other authorities. This open-air theatre is a little over an acre in extent, and is a valuable property. It had been leased to a restaurant keeper in the vicinity. Arrangements were made for the supply of light refreshments at bed-rock prices in the theatre, and other meals at low prices at the restaurant which is about fifty yards away. In addition a soldiers' club, managed by ladies, is equidistant, and at this comfortable resort refreshments are supplied in quiet rooms at low rates. Naturally the club has become a resort for all the soldiers in Cairo. Major Harvey, Commissioner of Police, has cleared the surrounding gardens of undesirable characters.

The club was placed under the management of a joint committee of which Her Excellency Lady MacMahon is Patroness, and Lady Maxwell is President. The executive committee consists of three members of the Y.M.C.A., and the expenses of managing the club were provided by the British Red Cross Society, Australian Branch, for the first three months. It was soon found that in order to make the club successful the athletic element must be developed, and splendid programmes were arranged—boxing, fencing, skating contests, and the like. The club provides writing-paper, games, war telegrams, Australian and other newspapers, shower baths, and other conveniences. As many as 1,500 soldiers are present on some of these occasions, and the club is visited by officers who periodically drop in amongst the men. Altogether the success has exceeded even the sanguine expectations of those who founded it.

The British Red Cross Society, Australian Branch, was most fortunate in securing such a site, as any one acquainted with the conditions of Cairo is fully aware.

The exact extent to which these clubs have contributed to the limitation of venereal disease cannot be accurately measured, but there is no doubt whatever in the minds of any one acquainted with the facts respecting their salutary and healthy influence. Under the new constitution of the Australian Red Cross money cannot be devoted to their maintenance, because it is not being used exclusively for the sick and wounded. Such is the ruling, although many convalescents use the clubs. It is regrettable that such a rigid ruling should have been established. It is absurd to permit men to become infected and then to assist them by doles of chocolate and tobacco, and yet to refuse to provide the necessary funds which assist so materially in preventing infection.

13. *Nurses' Rest Homes.*—The nurses in the hospitals had done excellent work under trying conditions, and it became obvious that many of them would break down unless holidays and rest were provided.

The British and Australian Red Cross Branches combined under the Presidency of Her Excellency Lady MacMahon, and opened two rest homes—one in Ramleh near the beach, and the other at Aboukir Bay, the site of Nelson's victory.

They were furnished by the Red Cross Societies and have been maintained by the Commonwealth Government so far as the Australian nurses are concerned. They have met a great want and have proved a boon and a blessing.

Conclusion.—The work has been very heavy and the circumstances far from easy. Taking everything into consideration and realising the pressure at both ends, the result can only be regarded as more than satisfactory. The policy of the Red Cross Society requires, however, some consideration.

The policy adopted until lately was that reasonable intimation should be given to the Red Cross Society of the requirements of those who want help. Under public pressure another policy may make its appearance—that of compelling the Red Cross Society to find out what people want. A word of caution is necessary. This policy

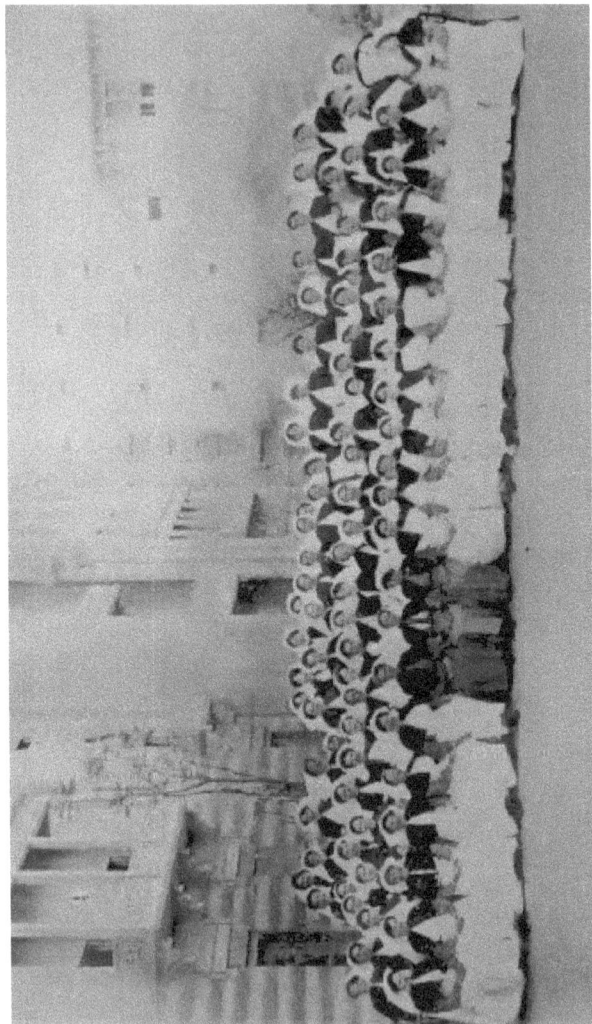

Matrons and Nurses, No. 1 Australian General Hospital.

will almost certainly result in the creation of an extensive business organisation and in the Red Cross undertaking much work which the government should do. In my opinion the Red Cross Society is entirely ancillary, its functions being to provide comforts and other things which the government cannot supply, and to act decisively at critical moments. It should, however, refrain from embarking on great national undertakings.

Everyone will endeavour to help the commissioners in their extensive and difficult task, and will look forward to the Australian Red Cross maintaining the high reputation which it has already gained amongst responsible officers in Egypt.

In conclusion it should be pointed out that during the whole period under review all necessary services were provided by the military authorities and the Red Cross was administered on military principles. Consequently there were no large expenses, no one received any money in payment for services, and the storage of goods was free.

If the Red Cross is to be administered on non-military lines many charges must be properly made and met, but the efficiency of the system instituted and now set aside must be judged largely from the standpoint of economic administration.

James W. Barrett,
Lieut.-Colonel.

(In this volume the original report forwarded to Melbourne has been expanded and amplified.)

Appendixes

1. Directions for the Conduct of the Red Cross Depot

Depot—conduct of.

1. The depot is placed under the charge of a medical officer who will have at his disposal nurses and orderlies in such numbers as the work from time to time may necessitate. Storage of goods.

2. All goods consigned to the Red Cross Depot shall be placed in store at once and rendered secure under lock and key at other than business hours.

Receipt Book.

3. All goods received will be entered in the Goods Receipt Book.

Requisitions—how dealt with

4. On receipt of requisitions signed by the officer commanding any unit, and countersigned by the officer commanding First Australian General Hospital, goods will be issued, and if necessary transport provided. Two clear lists shall be prepared on forms provided for the purpose, one to be receipted and returned to Red Cross Depot by the consignee and duplicate to be filed in office.

Stock-taking.

5. A Stock Book is to be kept showing the nature and quantity of material received, and the quantity distributed, so that at any time the stock remaining can be ascertained. This book to be checked once a month by stock-taking of the contents of the store and certified to by the M.O. in charge.

2. Result of Vote at No. 1 Auxiliary Convalescent Depot

The following items represent the wishes of 840 patients at Luna Park on July 29, 1915, ascertained by the O.C., Major Brown.

Four hundred and forty papers were received, a great number of patients failing to vote.

The patients were asked to make a list of twenty to thirty articles that would add to their comfort during their stay in hospital, and which could be supplied by a small fund at his disposal.

The average items on collected lists were 8.

Razors	249
Shaving-sticks	244
Razor strops	241
Tooth paste	221
Cigarettes	194
Toilet soap	188
Matches	170
Mirrors	177
Shaving-brushes	163
Tooth-brushes	148
Handkerchiefs	131
Tobacco	121
Pipes	106
Hairbrushes	99
Writing material	98
Haircombs	96
Fruit	63
Chocolate	54
Socks	37
Sweets	32
Pocket knives	30
Playing cards	21
Lead pencils	19
Housewives	14
Cigars	11
Biscuits	10
Walking-sticks	8
Shirts	8
Singlets	7
Belts	6
Tobacco pouches	4
Fountain pens	3
Bottles of ink	3
Nail brushes	3
Boot laces	3
Post cards	3
Mouth organs	3
Cigarette holder	1

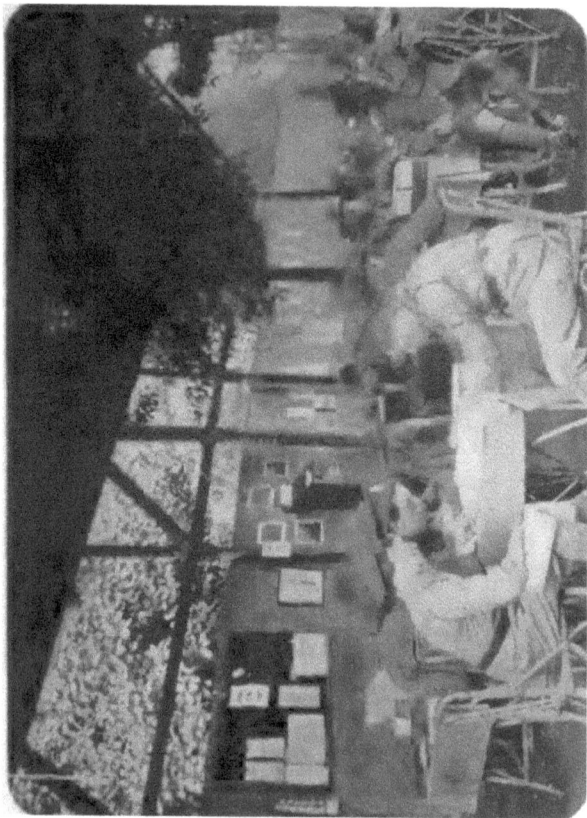

SOLDIERS' CLUB, ESBEKIEH, CAIRO.

Cigarette lighter	.	.	.	1
,, papers	.	.	.	1
Sponge .	.	.	.	1
Pair scissors	.	.	.	1
Soap box.	.	.	.	1
Nuts .	.	.	.	1
Dark eye-glasses	.	.	1 pair
Blades for safety razors	.	.	1 set
Notebook	.	.	.	1

3. Fence or Ambulance?

Some critics have objected to the Red Cross assisting Soldiers' Clubs. The following lines are commended to their notice. But for the Australian Branch British Red Cross there would have been no such Soldiers' Clubs as those provided at Esbekieh and Alexandria.

'Twas a dangerous cliff, as they freely confessed,
Though to walk near its crest was so pleasant;
But over its terrible edge there had slipped
A duke, and full many a peasant.
So the people said something would have to be done,
But their projects did not at all tally:
Some said, "Put a fence round the edge of the cliff";
Some, "an ambulance down in the valley."

But the cry for the ambulance carried the day,
For it spread through the neighbouring city,
A fence may be useful or not, it is true,
But each heart became brimful of pity
For those who had slipped over that dangerous cliff;
And the dwellers in highway and alley
Gave pounds or gave pence, not to put up a fence,
But an ambulance down in the valley.

"For the cliff is all right if you're careful," they said,
"And if folks even slip and are dropping,
It isn't the slipping that hurts them so much
As the shock down below when they're stopping."
So day after day, as those mishaps occurred,
Quick forth would these rescuers sally
To pick up the victims who fell off the cliff,
With the ambulance down in the valley.

Then an old sage remarked, "It's a marvel to me

145

That people give far more attention
To repairing results than to stopping the cause
When they'd much better aim at prevention.
Let us stop at its source all this mischief," cried he,
"Come, neighbours and friends, let us rally!
If the cliff we will fence we might almost dispense
With the ambulance down in the valley."

"Oh, he's a fanatic," the others rejoined.
"Dispense with the ambulance? Never!
He'd dispense with all charities, too, if he could!
No, no! We'll support them forever!
Aren't we picking folks up just as fast as they fall?
And shall this man dictate to us? Shall he?
Why should people of sense stop to put up a fence
While their ambulance works in the valley?"
But a sensible few, who are practical too,

Will not bear with such nonsense much longer;
They believe that prevention is better than cure,
And their party will soon be the stronger.
Encourage them, then, with your purse, voice, and pen,
And (while other philanthropists dally)
They will scorn all pretence, and put a stout fence
On the cliff that hangs over the valley.

Better guide well the young than reclaim them when old,
For the voice of true wisdom is calling:
"To rescue the fallen is good, but 'tis best
To prevent other people from falling.
Better close up the course of temptation and crime
Than deliver from dungeon or galley;
Better put a strong fence round the top of the cliff,
Than an ambulance down in the valley."

Joseph Malines.

THE RED CROSS POLICY: WANTED, A DEFINITION

Before leaving consideration of the details of the Red Cross question, attention should be directed to the numerous changes in the policy adopted by the British Red Cross Society, Australian Branch. No less than three different types of administration were rapidly adopted. It was first placed in the hands of Surgeon-General Williams and the

High Commissioner for Australia, in London; then it was placed under a committee in Egypt formed by the High Commissioner for Egypt, Sir Henry MacMahon, and six weeks later two commissioners were appointed to take the work over. Nothing more clearly illustrates the state of mental instability in which a first experience of war had thrown the population of Australia. The policy which was adopted by Surgeon-General Williams in connection with the Red Cross administration is that which we believe to be sound.

When acting as A.D.M.S. to the Australian Force in Egypt it became my duty (Lieut.-Col. Barrett) to sanction or modify the requisitions of medical stores for the various hospitals and units, and the instructions conveyed to me were that I could sanction any requisition provided that it was reasonable. If, however, it represented a new departure it must be authorised by the D.M.S. Egypt. This meant practically that everything could be obtained from Ordnance, and many of the Red Cross supplies became superfluous. That is to say, any necessary goods in the Red Cross store were utilised, but if they had not been there the government would have purchased them. In fact, it reduced the field in which the Red Cross could operate to comparatively small proportions. There is no doubt that, had it become necessary, I should have authorised the erection of shelter sheds and recreation huts in the various hospitals as a medical necessity. There was one advantage, and one advantage alone, in effecting these changes with the aid of the Red Cross. The action if sanctioned by superior officers could not be challenged by anyone else at the time, and could be effected with extraordinary speed.

I took the view that it was the business of the officer commanding the hospital, with the aid of the matron, sisters, and medical officers, to let me know what was thought necessary, and unless the requirement was outrageous it was immediately supplied. As a matter of fact no single request for money or goods was ever refused or seriously modified. Owing to pressure of public criticism another policy began to make its appearance. It was asserted that it was the duty of the Red Cross officer to visit the various hospitals to find out what the patients ought to receive. It will be seen that such a policy removed from the O.C.s of the hospitals, or any one to whom they may have delegated their powers, the responsibility for determining what patients should receive. Such a policy sooner or later must result in the creation of an army of people who are worrying to find out what they can do instead of being properly instructed by those responsible for the welfare of the patients.

It further tended to place in the hands of irresponsible people some control over the medical management of hospital cases. If lay visitors can enter a hospital and provide food for patients, they may next wish to provide drugs, etc. It seemed that the policy laid down in the first instance was sound, useful, and healthy.

When the commissioners took office they made a number of changes in detail. They shifted the position of the store; they printed different forms of requisition, and they took the goods out of the quartermaster's store and placed them in a store in the hospital, presided over by a volunteer. The goods were then obtained by requisition from the sisters and the matron. But as the President of the Red Cross Inquiry Court pointed out, with one trifling exception the method was not really altered. The control had simply ceased to be military, and had become civil. Consequently a large staff of capable people were withdrawn from their ordinary occupations in Australia, and devoted themselves to an administration which had been hitherto effected entirely by the soldiers.

We do not think that the change was right or desirable. It resulted in the creation of another body, not responsible directly to the military authorities, to do what is after all subsidiary work. The inevitable tendency will be for the Red Cross to take on function after function which should be undertaken by military authorities. The Red Cross is already supplying many articles which should be, and can be, supplied by Ordnance. For there is nothing that the Red Cross can supply that Ordnance cannot still more easily supply. It is quite true that the British Red Cross is managed on civil lines, and the British Red Cross supplies goods and does not supply money. But with a full knowledge of both systems we are strongly of opinion that the military method of management is in every respect preferable.

During the Red Cross Inquiry recently finished, to which allusion will be made elsewhere, day after day was necessarily spent by the court in endeavouring to decide what Red Cross should supply and what Ordnance should supply. What does it matter so long as the patient receives the articles? It does not concern him where they come from, and if the whole is under military control there is no need for this sharp and artificial line of demarcation. We are of opinion that in general the functions of the Red Cross should be to supply those additional comforts and accessories which make sick life more tolerable, to supply any goods which may be donated, and to make helpful donations of money in the way already indicated.

The presence in the store at Heliopolis of large quantities of goods—sheets, blankets, pillows, and the like—which could have been supplied by Ordnance, enabled us to rapidly tide over a great emergency. There is no doubt that the possession of money and goods by the Red Cross will prove of vast service in every campaign by reason of its emergency value. In fact the rapid expansion of No. 1 General Hospital during the crisis of May and June would not have proceeded with such smooth expedition had it not been for the large quantities of Red Cross stores which lay to hand and were instantly passed into the quartermaster's department. If, however, the supply had been under lay control, we can quite imagine circumstances in which argument, requisitions, forms, etc., might have seriously delayed operations.

Whilst on this subject reference must be made to the help afforded to the hospitals by Red Cross workers. Two schools of thought existed. Some commanding officers preferred to have no helpers, because of the trouble some of them gave. Others passed to the other extreme. Our own experience was that the workers organised by Mrs. Elgood were most helpful for the functions they undertook, with one or two exceptions, but those exceptional people gave a certain amount of trouble. They came not to help, but to criticise, and they carried their criticisms not to the commanding officer, but to the Australian public, and so caused trouble.

We are convinced that the Japanese method of organising the Red Cross is sound. It is organised and disciplined in time of peace, and when war is declared it becomes part of the army medical reserve and is mobilised for service. Everyone is under military control, and consequently these crudities are avoided. If we were to repeat our experience we should have welcomed the visitors, but insisted that they should be under some measure of discipline, and that a serious breach of regulations should be followed by their withdrawal. In some instances visitors wrote to the commander-in-chief, and complained of the food the patients were getting. The commander-in-chief sent the letters on to us, and we then brought the visitor in contact with the commanding officer of the hospital, and the complaint was investigated. How much more direct and simple it would have been if the visitor who saw something he believed to be wrong had immediately asked for the officer commanding! But the "secret and confidential" candid friend is apt to become somewhat of a pest.

There is another and more serious aspect of the matter. The medical officer is alone competent to judge what food should be issued to patients. Visitors who criticise the diet of the patient are assuming a function which they are obviously unable to discharge. Diet sheets are provided for each ward, and on these is entered the number of different diets prescribed by the medical officer. These diet sheets should be the only and the final authority of what should be issued to the patient in the way of eatables. As it happened, ladies sometimes brought into the different wards of the hospital foods which constituted an added danger to the patient. On one occasion green melons were issued to a large number of sick men by kind-hearted visitors. The men became so ill that the medical officer confiscated the melons, made inquiries, and only then ascertained the source of supply.

A strong-looking soldier on a milk diet might evoke the sympathies of a lady visitor, who lodged a complaint regarding the supply of food, but the nature of his disease and the method of treatment adopted by his medical officer are surely the principal consideration. As everything conceivable in the nature of food and drink can be supplied through these diet sheets, the obvious course is to pass all Red Cross foodstuffs directly into the quartermaster's department to be distributed in the ordinary, and the only safe, channel. This was the practice followed at Heliopolis.

The following articles were supplied in this way at the time of expansion, and show what assistance a properly controlled Red Cross system can render.

QUARTERMASTER'S REPORT

BY LIEUTENANT P. E. DEANE

ASSISTANCE RENDERED THE FIRST AUSTRALIAN GENERAL HOSPITAL BY RED CROSS IN HOSPITAL EXPANSION

April

Skating Rink opened.
Abbassia Venereal Diseases Hospital opened.
Casino Infectious   "   "   "

The following were obtained immediately on requisition on Red Cross:

Sheets	1,684
Pillowslips	2,300
Face washers	1,600
Towels	2,622
Handkerchiefs	1,000
Blankets	61
Pyjamas	489

Cotton shirts	701
Underpants	400
Socks	600
Flannel shirts	400
Slippers	67
Draw sheets	500
Pillows	69
Quilts	12
Old linen cases	2

May

Great rush of patients—Luna Park expanded, Palace Hotel expanded.

Patients admitted in four days from April 29 to May 2	1,543
Patients admitted during May	2,650

RED CROSS SUPPLIES

Sheets	1,381
Blankets	1,038
Towels	4,394
Pyjamas	1,176
Shirts	238
Handkerchiefs	500
Face washers	1,000

June

Rush of wounded continues. Atelier occupied, Sporting Club commenced.

Patients admitted during June	2,862

RED CROSS SUPPLIES

Pyjamas	790
Face washers	1,000
Sheets	900
Towels	1,500
Sponges	1,500
Handkerchiefs	1,500
Cotton shirts	950
Socks	1,000
Slippers	500

Pillowslips	1,000

Special hospital organised hurriedly by the department on June 17. Ras el Tin Convalescent Home, Alexandria.

RED CROSS SUPPLIES

Socks	1,000
Shirts	1,500
Pyjamas	750
Sheets	750
Blankets	750
Pillowslips	750
Face washers	1,500

July

Wounded still pour in. Sporting Club increased by addition of tennis court wards, Atelier and Luna Park accommodation increased.

Patients admitted in July	2,194

RED CROSS SUPPLIES

Sheets	2,000
Slippers	1,000
Pillowslips	3,400
Blankets	1,900
Shirts	2,000
Handkerchiefs	2,000
Towels	3,000
Socks	3,400
Face washers	3,000

August

Choubra Infectious Hospital hurriedly established and equipped by the department; 400-bed tent hospital added to Sporting Club.

RED CROSS SUPPLIES

Blankets	2,000
Cotton sheets	1,800
Towels	1,700
Handkerchiefs	2,400
Face washers	2,300
Socks	2,800
Pillowslips	214

CHAPTER 10

Suggested Reforms

The experience gained in connection with the establishment and extension of the First Australian General Hospital suggests modifications which should immensely increase efficiency. A base hospital modelled on the R.A.M.C. pattern may work exceedingly well in times of peace, or when staffed by R.A.M.C. or I.M.S. officers who have devoted their whole lives to the work. But base hospitals constructed during a great war, and staffed almost entirely with civilian elements the majority of whom are untrained in administration of any kind, do not work in all cases with the necessary degree of smoothness. It certainly does appear that changes in the base hospital establishment might be introduced with advantage.

In the first place there arises the question whether it is necessary for the commanding officer to be a medical practitioner, or whether, as in the case of the convalescent hospitals, he might be a combatant officer, or at all events a non-medical officer. The general consensus of opinion is that he should be a medical officer, though there is a great deal to be said on the other side. Almost the whole of his work is administrative, though he necessarily must have a good knowledge of clinical methods.

But unless such an officer be selected not simply with regard to seniority, but with regard to experience in administrative methods, and unless he be tactful and watchful, troubles are very likely to ensue. His task is beset with difficulties if he possesses character and insists on efficiency. Whatever doubt there may be, however, about the commanding officer, there need be none about many of the other positions.

A noteworthy feature of the First Australian General Hospital was the continual complaint from the medical officers that they had not come away to do administrative work. This distaste for administrative work was a constant source of trouble.

The registrar, as the principal executive officer of the hospital, whose business it is to carry out the decisions of the commanding officer, is at present invariably a medical officer. The greater part of his work does not need medical knowledge, and the difficulty might be obviated by the adoption of one of two methods. Either the registrar might be an educated business man or he might have such a one as his immediate understudy. In the latter event a very small portion of his day would be taken up with the duties of the registrar's office.

Similarly the orderly officer, whose business it is to deal with details concerning the rank and file, is usually a medical officer, and in some hospitals it is the practice to change this officer from day to day. At No. 1 General Hospital, however, his functions were so important that one medical officer was permanently told off to do this work. There is no doubt that the orderly officer need not be a medical officer, and might well be an invalided combatant officer, transferred to the army medical service.

Owing to modern developments another officer has made his appearance who is not provided for in any establishment—that is, the transport officer. Motor transport has become so large a portion of the work of the base hospital that a special officer is requisite for the purpose. There is no reason whatever why such an officer should be a medical man.

If these changes were made it would result in releasing at least three officers for clinical purposes.

The amount of clerical work that was necessitated by the returns furnished to the War Office, the Australian Government, Headquarters Egypt, and other departments was so great that a large staff of very competent clerks was required. The future establishment should certainly include not only a number of trained stenographers, but someone versed in statistical work. The lessons to be learned are so numerous and so important that something of the kind should be done. Furthermore, in the quartermaster's department there was a demand not only for stenographers, but for men who had been accustomed to the methodical ways of a large warehouse.

Were all these changes made there is no doubt that the efficiency of the administration would be increased and the burden of the work lightened.

As regards clinical work other desirable changes might be made.

Senior men who have been in full practice, and who come to a base hospital as physicians or surgeons with the rank of lieutenant-colonel, are apt to be entrusted with the detailed administration of medical or surgical wards. They are often unfitted by training for such administration and are frequently disinclined to undertake the work. It would be far better to leave the actual detailed administration of the wards in the hands of a comparatively junior man with the rank of major, and to retain these senior officers as consultants only.

Consultants of course possess great powers, since their authority as regards the clinical work itself is absolute. They can do as much or as little as they like, but they are in complete control and are absolutely responsible for the treatment of the cases. Our own feeling is that in such a position they would be far more comfortable and would be more efficient.

On the subject of specialists there is much to be said. It is almost incredible that a base hospital should have been formed without being provided with an ophthalmic and aural specialist. The change has been made since war began, but it seems inconceivable that any one should have contemplated the efficient handling of wounds and diseases without such aid. At the First General Hospital the ophthalmic and aural department was the largest and most heavily worked department in the hospital, partly owing to the fact that one of us had been appointed Consulting Oculist to the Forces in Egypt, and that much of the work consequently centred at Heliopolis.

Similarly the failure of the Australian Government to provide dentists in the first instance is difficult to understand. The day has gone by when it is possible to exclude from the force a man who possesses dentures or defective teeth, and it is practically impossible to complete the work for the recruits before they leave. So it became necessary at No. 1 General Hospital to borrow two dentists from the New Zealand Government, to fit them out with Red Cross money and goods, and in this way to meet informally the difficulty. Subsequently the Australian Government appointed a corps of dentists, and the problem was to some extent solved, though even now the demand far exceeds the supply. There is no doubt that dentists are wanted not only at the base hospitals, but also near the firing line, as the dispatch of a man from the firing line to the base hospital to obtain dental treatment represents a waste of time and money.

It is further desirable to attach one or more anaesthetists to every hospital.

It must, however, be said that the constant changes of staff which took place at No. 1 Hospital owing to the various exigencies of the military situation rendered it extremely difficult to keep a physician or surgeon in any fixed position for any length of time. Consequently a certain amount of pliability and adaptability was absolutely necessary. At the same time, if the organisation were sketched in the manner indicated, the problem would have been more simple, and good results easier to obtain.

There is no doubt that one medical officer (who could be attached to the Pathological Laboratory in addition to the Clinical Pathologist) should devote himself entirely to sanitary work. This duty is not taken too seriously, and should be emphasised. It would really be better to rename this officer the "Prophylactic Officer," unless a better term can be found, and it should be his aim and duty, not simply to enforce cleanliness, but to actively exert himself to ward off disease.

Stress may be laid on the usefulness of a sensible chaplain, whose value depends on his own interpretation of his duties. The chaplain (Colonel Kendrew) at No. 1 General Hospital not only attended to the religious needs of men, but earned their affection and respect by managing the extensive post office and library, the canteen, and by helping with Red Cross work. It is just these badly defined functions in a base hospital which a chaplain can discharge so well.

We think also that women might be used in base hospitals as stenographers, ward maids, telephone operators, and the like. Base hospitals in the future are not likely to be housed in tents, and under rough conditions. At present, trained nurses are sent to the Stationary Hospitals. It seems a pity to waste fine young men, who could be combatants, as orderlies in a base hospital.

Masseurs are certainly badly wanted in a base hospital, and it is difficult to understand the objection to their incorporation. The difficulty was removed in Egypt by employing Egyptians.

Electricians, i.e. orderlies who in civil life are electricians, are required in every base hospital, and at Heliopolis they were invaluable for general purposes, and as aids to the radiographer. They should, however, form part of the establishment, and should number two or three.

Is it not clear that chefs, laundrymen, skilled carpenters, and other tradesmen are also required?

The table which follows represents the establishment of the ordinary 520-bed hospital, R.A.M.C. It has been adopted by Australia, but the Australian establishment allows for 93 nurses instead of 43. If the foregoing suggestions are adopted, as we think they should be, this table would require material alteration.

A GENERAL HOSPITAL (520 BEDS)

WAR ESTABLISHMENTS

DETAIL.	PERSONNEL.					
	Officers.	W.O.	St. Sergts. and Sergts.	Buglers.	Rank and File.	Total.
Lieut.-Col. in charge .	1	—	—	—	—	1
Lieut.-Cols.　.　　.	2	—	—	—	—	2
Majors—						
Sec. and Registrar .	1	—	—	—	—	1
General Duties　.	4	—	—	—	—	4
Captains or Subs.　.	12	—	—	—	—	12
Quartermaster .　　.	1	—	—	—	—	1
Warrant Officers　.	—	2	—	—	—	2
Sergeants—						
Nursing Duties　.	—	—	4	—	—	4
Steward　　.　.	—	—	1	—	—	1
Dispenser　.　.	—	—	2	—	—	2
Cook　.　.　.	—	—	1	—	—	1
Pack Storekeeper .	—	—	1	—	—	1
Linen　　,,　.	—	—	1	—	—	1
Clerks .　.　.	—	—	3	—	—	3
Buglers　.　.　.	—	—	—	2	—	2
Corporals—						
Steward　.　.	—	—	—	—	1	1
Cook　.　.　.	—	—	—	—	1	1
Clothing Storekeeper	—	—	—	—	1	1
General Duties　.	—	—	—	—	1	1
Supernumeraries　.	—	—	—	—	3	3
Privates—						
Steward's Stores　.	—	—	—	—	2	2
Cooks　.　.　.	—	—	—	—	3	3
Pack Stores .　.	—	—	—	—	1	1
Linen　　,,　.	—	—	—	—	1	1
Clothing ,,　.	—	—	—	—	1	1
Clerks .　.　.	—	—	—	—	2	2
Ward duties .　.	—	—	—	—	66	66
Batman　.　.	—	—	—	—	25	25
General Duties　.	—	—	—	—	11	11
Supernumeraries　.	—	—	—	—	6	6
TOTAL　.　.	21	2	13	2	126	164

With reference to the duties of N.C.O.s and men, nothing gave more trouble than the fact that men recruited in Australia were made N.C.O.s before their special qualifications were known. There is no officer in the army whose position is so thoroughly safeguarded as the N.C.O., and nothing but the adverse decision of a court martial can effect his removal. Yet an unsuitable and even dangerous man, from the point of view of the sick, may do nothing to warrant a court martial (which no one enjoys). These appointments should be made therefore with great care. Such considerations, of course, lead to but one conclusion, *viz.* the necessity for sketching out these hospitals in time of peace. Scratch enlistments are too dangerous.

The "grouser" is always with us, and sometimes gives trouble. The particular Australian "grouse" was that the Australian hospitals should have been nearer the front than Cairo, and at last No. 3 Australian General Hospital was placed at Mudros.

Now we have always understood that a large base hospital cannot be placed far from a great city. A city grows in a particular place for natural reasons—water supply, lighting, transit, etc. The hospital gets the benefit of all these agencies, whereas it was necessary at Lemnos to create them. The result was somewhat disastrous as regards supplies, and might have been foreseen.

"Grousers" should stay at home, and exercise their privileges there.

The difficulties of obtaining supplies by requisition were easily surmounted at Heliopolis because of the broad policy adopted by the officer commanding the Australian Intermediate Base, Colonel Sellheim, C.B.

Ordnance cannot supply the varied requirements of a group of expert medical officers during a great war, and delays cause untold annoyance to active men. On the other hand, it would never do to give the staff a free hand to purchase when and how it pleased.

The institution of "local purchase orders" met the difficulty. The O.C. of the hospital sent in a requisition for something which could not be obtained from Ordnance, marking it "urgently required." The A.D.M.S. endorsed it, or, if it were an entirely new line, asked the D.M.S. to endorse it. The Ordnance officer then issued a local purchase order to the medical officer, who made the purchase. The method combined a measure of control with reasonable speed in execution.

We have no sympathy with the usual references to military redtape. If the administration is competent, the military system is thor-

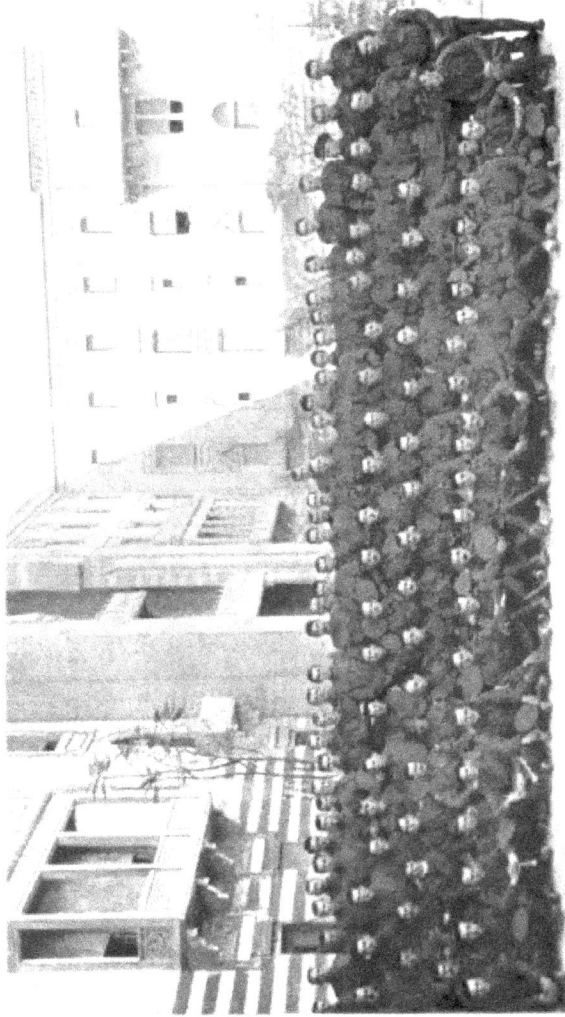

N.C.O.s AND MEN, No. 1 AUSTRALIAN GENERAL HOSPITAL.

oughly sound from the business point of view, and from the standpoint of record difficult to improve on. It may be at times a little cumbersome, but it is much easier to fall in with it than to attempt to effect alteration during war. We never had any real difficulty with requisitions, although supplies were sometimes withheld from us on grounds of policy not disclosed at the moment.

There is no doubt that the erratic changes of staff were injurious. Some medical officers preferred the front, others the base, and an attempt was made to effect an orderly system of periodical exchange. Orders, however, were continually arriving to send so many medical officers, so many nurses, and so many orderlies, here and there, with the result that at the end of ten months the original medical staff had disappeared, many of the nurses were new, and so were most of the orderlies. Whenever there was a shortage of staff near the front, the base hospitals were depleted. These changes were inevitable in the circumstances, but they emphasised the value of the advice given by Colonel Manifold, that there cannot be too many unattached junior medical officers in a campaign. The following report from Major Brown, Officer Commanding Luna Park No. 1 Auxiliary Hospital, shows what he experienced owing to these oscillations:

First Australian General Hospital, Luna Park

April 30	. Opened with 296 patients	
May 2 .	. 790 patients	Staff : 4 sisters, 4 orderlies, and myself. With Captains Bentley, McDonald, and White from Light Horse Regiments.
May 6 .	.	Sisters increased to 13.
May 14 .	. 1,171 patients	13 sisters, 4 medicos, and 40 orderlies (mostly untrained).
May 18 .	. 1,244 patients	
June 7 .	. 1,099 patients (also 65 Casino)	41 sisters (new).
June 9 .	. 1,370 patients (also 65 Casino)	,, ,, ,,
June 11 .	. 1,620 patients (also 65 Casino)	,, ,, ,,

160

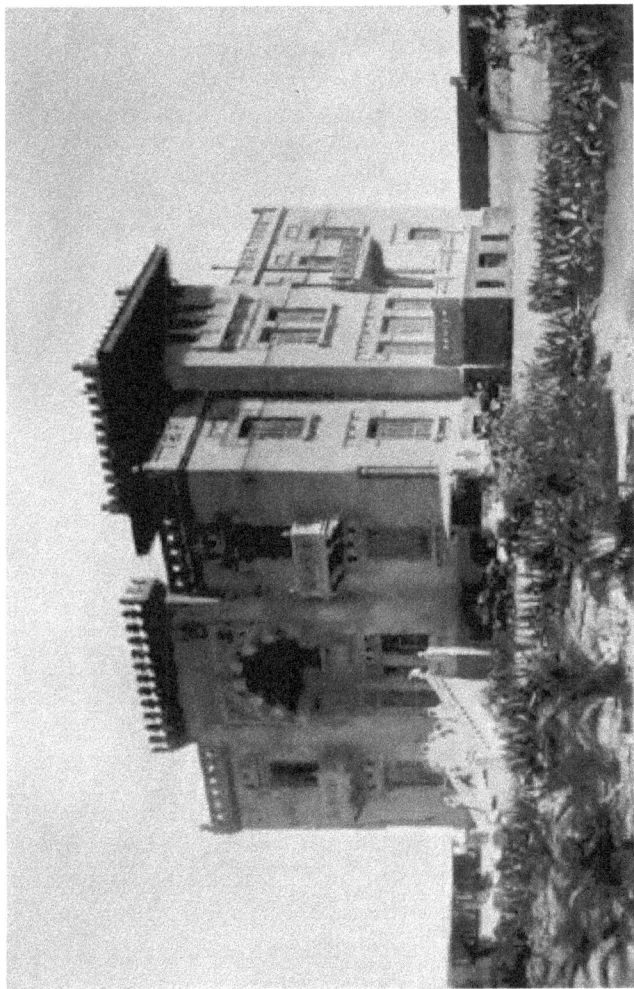

PALACE OF PRINCE IBRAHIM KHALIM (NURSES' HOME).

| June 16 . | . 1,520 patients | Still 4 medical officers, Capt. Brown, Capt. Single, Capt. Love-grove, and Capt. Craig. |
| June 17 . | . | Medical officers now in-creased ; sisters also increased. |

With reference to orderlies, the work from May 3 has been done with 10 A.M.C. men and 30 men drawn from the patients.

On June 17, 40 reinforcement A.M.C. men were detailed for duty. Up to June 16 over 1,600 patients have been discharged. On May 23 the Operating Theatre was opened.

For the 1,600 patients we had six cooks with six natives to assist.

T. F. Brown, Captain,
Officer in Charge, Luna Park.

Heliopolis,
June 17, 1915.

Of the 93 nurses belonging to the hospital, within a week of land-ing no fewer than 47 were taken away and dispatched to various parts of Egypt, *viz*.:

Port Said (Clearing Hospital)	21
Pont de Koubbeh (Egyptian Army H.)	9
The Citadel (British Hospital	6
Alexandria	2
Transport duty	8
Returned to Australia (sick)	1
	47

No. 1 Australian General Hospital was much inspected by keen and curious, as well as sympathetic, eyes. His Highness the *Sultan*, Their Excellencies Sir Henry and Lady MacMahon, the General Of-ficer Commanding-in-Chief, Egypt, the General Officer Command-ing Australian and New Zealand Army Corps, and many other distin-guished people honoured the hospital by an inspection.

The following letters were written by three distinguished visitors. Two Corps Orders are also attached.

Shepheard's Hotel, Cairo,
May 20, 1915.

Dear Colonel Ramsay Smith,

Allow me to congratulate you upon the admirable medical arrangements at Heliopolis, and upon the excellent hospital you have established there. One is at first disposed to say, 'How well the building adapts itself to a hospital!' until the true fact becomes revealed of the genius displayed in converting a decidedly refractory building into a place for the sick. You and your staff have done wonders and have once more shown that in the land of Egypt *it is possible to make bricks without straw.*

Australia may well be proud of the part she has played in this war, and I can pay no higher compliment than by saying that the medical arrangements of the Australian Army are as splendid as are the fighting qualities of its men.

Above all I was impressed with the energy and enthusiasm with which the work at Heliopolis is being carried on, with the ingenuity and resource displayed at every turn, and with the thoroughness that was manifest in every department of the vast hospital.

The generosity with which Australia has provided motor ambulances for the whole country and Red Cross stores for everyone, British or French, who has been in want of same is beyond all words.

I only hope that the people of Australia will come to know of the splendid manner in which their wounded have been cared for, and of the noble and generous work which the great colony has done under the banner of the Red Cross.

Yours sincerely,
(Signed) Frederick Treves.

Turf Club, Cairo,
June 21, 1915.

Dear Colonel Ramsay Smith,

I am just off to the Dardanelles, and then back to Cairo, but I felt that I must write and thank you for your kindness in sending me those excellent and interesting photographs, which I shall treasure, and the memory of the interesting day I spent with you at your wonderful hospital. I also thank you for your report and for the copy of Sir F. Treves's letter.

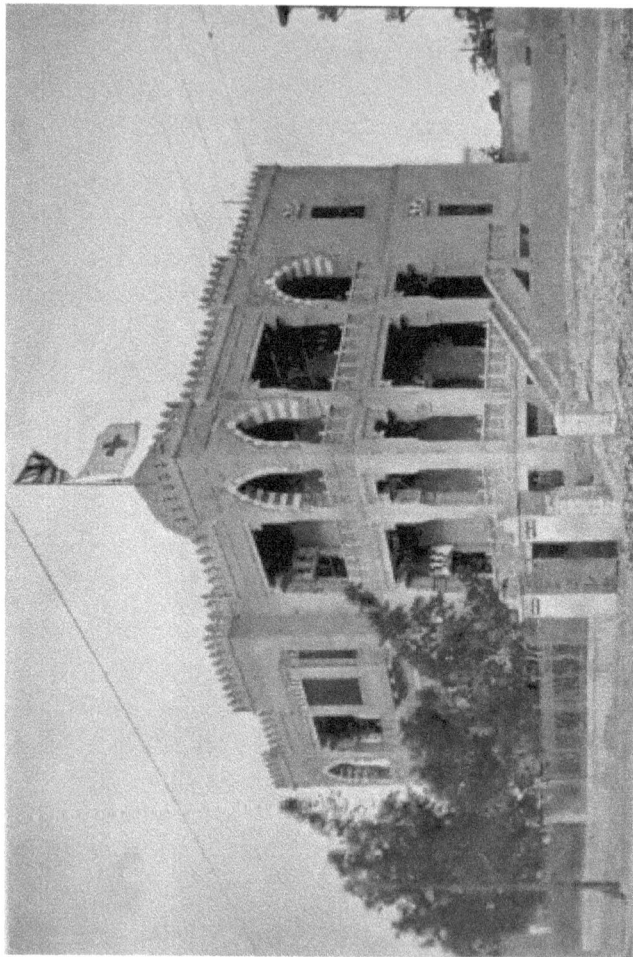

GORDON HOUSE, HELIOPOLIS (NURSES' HOME).

You must feel proud of your work at Heliopolis, on which I heartily congratulate you. It is a monument of skill in administration and the surmounting of what would at first appear to be insurmountable difficulties.

Hoping soon to see you again,

Yours very sincerely,

(Signed) A. W. Mayo-Robson.

St. Mark's Buildings, Alexandria,
June 5, 1915.

Dear Major Barrett,

I have been away at the front or I should have written to you sooner to thank you for the interesting visit which you enabled Sir Frederick Treves and myself to pay to your hospital and stores. I enclose an extract of a report which I made on May 25 to the Hon. Arthur Stanley, Chairman of the British Red Cross Society and Order of St. John in London.

You may have noticed a minute published in the press with the approval of the G.O.C., Sir John Maxwell, in which it was laid down that all Red Cross work, except the Australian Red Cross work, should be under the control of the British Red Cross and Order of St. John. I hope you will not think that in drafting this minute in this way I wished to convey that we were not working in perfect harmony with your Red Cross, but I feel that we could hardly suggest to you that you should be in any way under our control. At the same time, I hope that when you either come here, or when I come back to Cairo, that we may have an opportunity of conferring together so that we may so co-ordinate as far as possible our mutual work.

May I add that I went to the Dardanelles in a transport with over a thousand of your brave soldiers, many of whom were returning to the Peninsula after having already been wounded. It is impossible to speak too highly of their gallantry, and of the splendid spirit they displayed. I need not tell you that I heard of their fighting qualities at the front, since their heroic deeds in this campaign have already become a matter of history.

Yours sincerely,

(Signed) Courtauld Thomson,

Chief Commissioner for British Red Cross and Order of St. John, Malta, Egypt, and Near East Commission.

Extract from a Report from Lieut.-Colonel Sir Courtauld Thomson, Chief Commissioner of the British Red Cross and Order of St. John, to the Hon. Arthur Stanley, dated May 25, 1915.

A striking feature in Cairo is the remarkable work which is being done by the Australian Red Cross. They have not only two exceptionally large hospitals and the large convalescent home, but they supply the motor transport for the wounded for the whole of Egypt. They have also very large Red Cross stores which they have brought with them. With these articles they have been more than generous, and I am informed that they have given away to the hospitals for our own troops something like 75 *per cent.* of whatever they had.

Extract from Corps Orders, March 28, 1915

Appreciation.—The D.M.S. Egypt, who visited the hospital yesterday afternoon, has requested the officer commanding to convey to the officers, nurses, N.C.O.s, and men in the hospital his appreciation of the work done and the thorough character of the organisation.

Extract from Corps Orders, May 1, 1915

Appreciation.—The D.M.S. Egypt, Surgeon-General Ford, witnessed the detraining of the invalids who arrived here Wednesday evening. He asked Major Barrett to convey to the officer commanding his great appreciation of the excellence of the arrangements and the efficient and quiet manner in which the work was done.

He congratulates officers and men on the splendid work they are doing and requests that it shall be communicated to them in Corps Orders.

Looking back, does it not seem essential that these hospitals should have been formed, at all events in outline, in time of peace? That their commanding officers and essential staff should have been marked out beforehand, so that on the declaration of war the gaps could have been filled in from the reserve without difficulty? Satisfactory appointments are much less likely to be made in the turmoil which follows the declaration of war than in the atmosphere of deliberate calm which prevails in time of peace. Had such an arrangement prevailed, the First

Australian General Hospital would certainly never have been recruited from three States distant from one another hundreds of miles.

Finally, Australian hospitals in time of war should either be regarded as responsible solely to the Australian military authorities and government, or handed over without reserve to the R.A.M.C., and placed entirely under the control of the British authorities. Where two different authorities exist, as in the case of the First General Hospital, a large amount of trouble and delay is almost certain to ensue. The adoption of the latter course is in our judgment absolutely essential if efficiency is to be secured.

As is invariably the case, weaknesses in any system are only revealed by costly experience. But while in the Australian Medical Service the experience need not have been so costly, we can at least profit by what has occurred, and frame a stronger and a better policy for the future.

On the whole, the record of work done in most trying circumstances is, we think, satisfactory. It is true that the universal democratic fault was evidenced in the lack of preparation for conditions which were fairly obvious. Nevertheless the adaptability and growth of the hospitals in time of great emergency were achievements of the highest order.

Yet it would be unwise to leave the subject with the usual Anglo-Saxon expression of satisfaction that the crisis was passed. The history reviewed has too deep a significance. It must be regarded not merely as an individual incident, but as an indication of the inefficiency evidenced by too many departments of the Empire.

The causes which found the medical services unprepared, which forced them to expand to the breaking-point, and which led to the criticism of the hospital authorities, are not departmental or sectional—they are national. If attacks on individuals are permitted, initiative will be stifled; if on the other hand we are content to follow the time-worn policy of "muddling through," the virile people who skirt the border lines of our Empire will sooner or later bid us make way for stronger men.

Our policy for the future must be one of scientific organisation and calculated preparation in every department. We must not only appoint capable administrators, but also trust them. We can again, if we like, obtain that temporary mental tranquillity which comes to a democracy—and to an ostrich—which does not or will not see the calamity which threatens it, but temporary beatitude will be purchased at the price of an empire. Never was it more certainly true that the price of liberty is eternal vigilance.

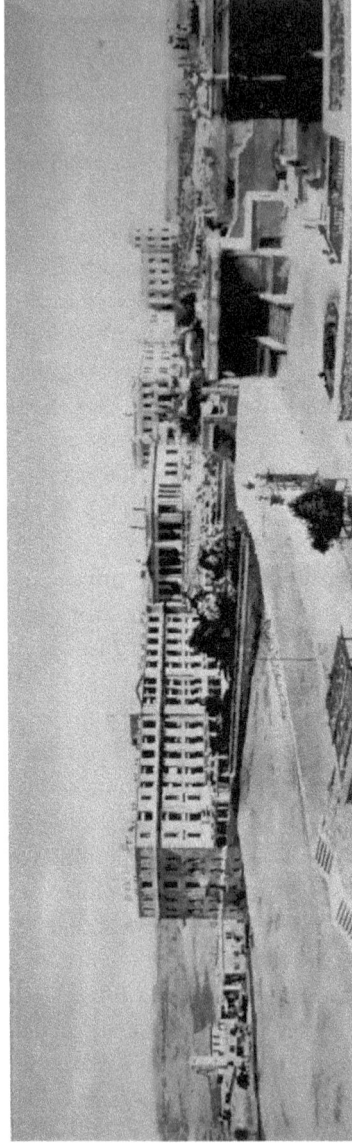

AUSTRALIAN CONVALESCENT HOSPITAL, AL HAYAT, HELOUAN.

Chapter 11

Postscript

One of us (J. W. B.) was invalided to England in the middle of November 1915, and returned to Egypt at the end of March 1916.

He resigned his commission in the Australian Army Medical Corps on February 28, and was appointed temporary Lt.-Col. in the R.A.M.C. on February 29. On his return to Egypt he was appointed Consulting Aurist to the Forces in Egypt, and was a member of the Council of the British Red Cross Society and of the Y.M.C.A. He consequently had an opportunity of witnessing the termination of many of the arrangements for which he had been in part originally responsible, and desires to make brief reference to them.

No. 1 Australian General Hospital with its many off-shoots, including the four auxiliary hospitals and the venereal disease hospital, was located in Egypt for periods of twelve to eighteen months. No. 2 Australian General Hospital was in Egypt about fourteen months. Yet it was stated that each and every one of these hospitals when established were to be temporarily located in Egypt for a few weeks. Luna Park, *i.e.* No. 1 Auxiliary Hospital, was in existence approximately sixteen months. An enormous number of sick and wounded, said to be 18,000, was passed through it with an infinitesimal death-rate, viz. four or five persons.

Since the end of 1915, the No. 3 Australian General Hospital was moved from Mudros to the Barracks at Abbassia, Cairo. The expenditure necessary to fit the barracks for the reception of No. 3 Australian General Hospital and the time taken are very interesting, since they show how utterly impossible any such arrangement would have been during the inrush of wounded in 1915. Stress is laid on the value of auxiliary hospitals as the only practicable means of surmounting difficulties at that time, in the report of the Committee of Inquiry into the

Administration of the Australian Branch British Red Cross in Egypt.

Looking back at the practical conclusion of the work of the Australian Army Medical Corps in Egypt, it is quite evident that the policy originally adopted was the only one possible in the circumstances, and the results have fully justified it.

THE FLY CAMPAIGN

Very active steps were taken during 1916 in the direction of a campaign for the destruction of flies. The only addition that need be made to previous remarks is reference to the ingenious fly traps which have been devised. A large one was designed by Lt.-Col. Andrew Balfour, C.M.G., and is described the journal of the Army Medical Corps of July 1916. A modified form of this trap, furnished by the British Red Cross in Egypt, costs about 16s., and was most effective. These traps have been known to catch as many as 20,000 flies a day.

The smaller trap, which can be used indoors, and is made of zinc gauze, was made in large quantities by the British Red Cross Society in Alexandria, and distributed throughout Egypt.

Another kind of trap, a Japanese invention, with clockwork mechanism, manufactured by Owari Tokei, Kabushiki, Kwaisha, Japan, has also been very successful. As many as 3,000 flies have been captured in one instance in an hour. It has a considerable advantage over the other traps in that its mechanism interests everyone.

Like all fly traps, however, the utility of these devices depends upon placing them in the hands of men whose business it is to see that they are properly baited and cared for, and on some ingenuity with regard to the baits. For the larger traps placed out-of-doors the best baits were found to be fishes' heads or the entrails of fowls, whilst the best bait for the smaller indoor trap was a mixture of beer or whisky and sugar.

It is, of course, quite evident that the destruction of flies by traps is not logically sound, since the proper method of control of the fly pest is by the destruction of all refuse; but as that is impracticable in Egypt, the traps were of great assistance.

In 1916 the fly pest as usual became marked during two periods in the year; viz. at the beginning and the end of summer. At the height of summer the dryness and desiccation evidently prevent the breeding of flies, a fact to be borne in mind in Australia.

The returns given in the House of Commons respecting the Gallipoli Campaign place the casualties at 116,000, and the cases invalided at 96,000. As a very large number of the cases of the sick were due to intestinal infections, some idea of the damage which may be caused by flies can be imagined.

The discovery of *bilharzia* eggs and the organisms of dysentery and diarrhoea in the faeces of flies made it clear that the fly plays an even larger part in disseminating disease than has hitherto been understood. It really would appear that if the flies were destroyed infective diseases would fall to small proportions.

THE VENEREAL-DISEASE PROBLEM

The venereal-disease problem in the early part of 1916 gave very great concern, and active measures were taken to deal with it. In spite of all the ameliorating influences the problem reached its most serious phase in March and April 1916, as questions put in the House of Commons show (*vide Lancet*, April 8, 1916). I think I express the conviction of certainly 90 *per cent.* of medical men in stating that nothing but education and educated prophylaxis will ever enable us to get rid of this source of destruction.

Y.M.C.A. AND RED CROSS

The Soldiers' Club in the Ezbekieh Garden grew in favour and was extended in area and staff. In the autumn of 1915 some ladies became available, and did splendid service in the superintendence of the catering for the men in the Club, and by their presence there did much to help.

A more extended experience of the work of the Y.M.C.A. and of the Red Cross has given much cause for thought. The Y.M.C.A. organisation appears to me to be excellent, since it is the organisation which caters for the social welfare of the soldier, wherever he may be, whether in camp or at the base; and the work is conducted by men whose business it is to understand him and see that all reasonable wants are gratified. In Egypt as I write (July 1916) there are no fewer than forty-seven Y.M.C.A. huts and centres, and Y.M.C.A. officers in the desert, in the oases, and elsewhere, doing their very best to make the soldiers comfortable. In other words, the business of the Y.M.C.A. is to provide comfort by personal service over and above military necessaries for the men who are well.

The Red Cross Society, on the other hand, attends to the wants of the sick and wounded, and its functions have already been discussed. They may, however, be supplemented by the following definition of the work of the Red Cross which was furnished by the High Commissioner for Egypt, Sir Henry MacMahon:

> Government supplies all the necessities for the care, treatment, and transport of the sick and wounded, while the Red Cross supplements these necessities by everything that can in any way go to the comfort and well-being of the sick and wounded soldiers. The distinction between necessities and comforts is sometimes so indefinite that the Red Cross, wherever possible, endeavours to have both ready to hand for use when needed.

And later:

> A word must be said here about the work of the Red Cross Stores. The object of the Red Cross has never been to supply in any large quantities the goods which the War Office sends to the wounded, but it does its best to provide the troops with such things as the War Office does not supply at all or cannot supply at a given time. A State Department, bound as it rightly is by hard-and-fast rules, cannot work as quickly as a private body with more elastic regulations; moreover, the supplies of any department may change at times, hence it happens that the British Red Cross occasionally supply certain things more than the War Office can, or it may supplement the War Office supplies, and it does so until the War Office steps in again. Further, the Red Cross supplies many things or small luxuries which the authorities cannot possibly supply, and these are just the things which are most appreciated by the sick and wounded.

In other words, the function of the Red Cross is to assist over and above necessity, and to be ready to act in event of emergency.

The following lists of the Australian Branch and Egyptian Branch of the British Red Cross show that in both cases, but particularly in the case of the Australian Branch, the Red Cross is supplying articles which should clearly be supplied by government. There is considerable danger in allowing this system to become too largely developed. In the first place in the case of the Red Cross there is no rigid system of accountancy such as military regulation requires, and the natural tendency for commanders will be to get goods in the easiest possible manner; nevertheless, it may not be the best thing for the service.

The British Red Cross safeguards the practice more fully than the younger branch, and its lead might well be followed. (See lists following)

AUSTRALIAN BRANCH BRITISH RED CROSS SOCIETY

LIST OF ARTICLES IN RED CROSS STORES WHICH MUST BE REQUISITIONED FOR BY COMMANDING OFFICERS OF UNITS FOR THE CARE OF THE SICK AND WOUNDED AND WHERE THERE IS NO RED CROSS STORE.

To the Commissioners,
    Australian Branch British Red Cross Society,
        Shepheard's Hotel, Cairo.

Please send to..................................... ....
the following articles :

Quantity	Description
	Clothing
	Balaclava Caps
	Cardigans
	Cholera Belts
	*Cushions, Air
	* ,, Ordinary
	Dressing Gowns
	Facewashers
	Fly Veils
	Gloves
	*Handkerchiefs
	Mittens
	*Mosquito Nets
	*Slippers, Hospital
	*Socks
	* ,, Bed
	*Surgeons' Aprons
	* ,, Caps
	* ,, Gowns
	* ,, Swabs
	*Towels
	* ,, Glass
	Underpants, Cotton
	,, Flannel
	Undershirts, Cotton
	,, Flannel
	Foodstuffs
	Allenbury's Diet
	,, Food
	Arrowroot

Quantity	Description
	Clothing—continued
	Mufflers
	*Pillows
	*Pillow Slips
	Pneumonia Jackets
	*Pyjamas, Cotton
	* ,, Flannel
	*Quilts
	*Sheets
	*Shirts, Cotton
	* ,, Flannel
	* ,, Hospital
	*Shoes, Deck
	Lime Juice
	Linseed Meal
	Malt Extract
	Oatmeal
	Pickles
	Plum Puddings
	Port Wine
	Robinson's Barley
	,, Groats
	Semolina
	Soda Water
	Sweets
	Tapioca
	Tinned Rabbits
	,, Tomatoes
	,, Tripe
	,, Vegetables

Beef Extract
Benger's Food
Biscuits
Bovril
Brandy
Ceregen
Chocolate
Cocoa
Cocoa-and-Milk
Coffee Essence
Coffee-and-Milk
Condensed Milk
Cornflour
Cornina
Fruits, Dried
   ,,   Tinned
Glaxo
Horlick's M. Milk
Jam
Jelly Crystals
Lactogen

*Hospital Basins
*Hot-water Bottles
 Housewives
*Insectibane
 Looking-glasses
 Matches
*Medicine Glasses
 Old Linen
*Oil Heaters
 Pencils
 Periodicals
 Pipes
*Primus Stoves
*Razors
*Razor Strops
*Rubber Sheeting

General

*Absorbent Wool
*Bandages
*Bed Cradles
* ,, Rests
* ,, Screens
 Books
*Brushes, Hair
* ,,   Nail
* ,,   Tooth
*Camp Stools
 Cigarettes
*Combs
*Crutches
*Deck Chairs
 Eau-de-Cologne
 Envelopes
 Fly Veils
 Fly Whisks
 Gramophone
   Needles

*Safety Pins
*Smoked Glasses
*Soap, Monkey
  Brand
*Soap, Shaving
* ,, Toilet
*Splints
*Sponges
*Tables, Folding
*Thermometers
 Tobacco
*Toilet Paper
 Tooth Paste
*Vaseline
 Writing Pads

Note A.—As a general rule the Commissioners only supply goods that cannot be obtained from either Ordnance Dept. Army Service Corps, or Base Medical Depot Stores. Any O.C. requisitioning for goods of a kind properly obtainable from those sources should state on the requisition that the goods applied for cannot be obtained from the usual source.

Note B.—Regimental Medical Officers can obtain their requirements from the O.C. of the nearest Field Ambulance, who will
forward requisitions to Red Cross.

. . . .
Officer in charge of Hospital.

[All the articles marked * were permanent Government
issues, and any of the foodstuffs would have been supplied
by Government if necessary. There was no practical difficulty
in obtaining any articles from Government on proper application being made.]

BRITISH RED CROSS AND ORDER OF ST. JOHN

No. of Patients . . . .   *For the Use of Patients*

LIST OF ARTICLES IN RED CROSS STORES WHICH MAY BE
REQUISITIONED FOR.

————————————————191

To the Commissioner,
    British Red Cross and Order of St. John,
        Gresham Buildings, Cairo.

Please send to . . . .
the following articles :

Quantity	Description	Quantity	Description
B.D.M.S.	Air Beds (Rubber)	O.D.	Caps
	Air Rings (Rubber)	O.D.	Cardigans
B.D.M.S.	Air Cushions (Rubber)		Carrying Chairs
	Ash Trays		Cholera Belts
	Balaclava Helmets		Chocolate
B.D.M.S.	Bandages	A.S.C.	Cigarettes
	Bandage Winders		Cloths (Pantry and Kitchen)
B.D.M.S.	Bellows (for Air Beds)	O.D.	Combs
O.D.	Bed Pans	B.D.M.S.	Cotton Wool
O.D.	Bed Rests	B.D.M.S.	Crutches
O.D.	Bed Trays		Dressing Gowns
	Bed Jackets		Dressings
	Bed Pockets		Deck Chairs
O.D.	Blankets		Eau-de-Cologne
	Blacking		Face Flannels
B.D.M.S.	Boric Lint		Face Nets
	Books and Magazines	O.D.	Fans
		O.D.	Fly Whisks
			Fly Veils
	Boot Brushes		Food Slicers

175

A.S.C.	Bovril	O.D.	Feeding Cups
	Biscuits		Games
	Brandy	B.D.M.S.	Gauze Tissue
O.D.	Camp Stools		Goulas
	Gramophones	B.D.M.S.	Rubber Gloves
	Hair Brushes	O.D.	Shaving Brushes
O.D.	Handkerchiefs		Soap (Toilet)
	Head Shields		Spirits
O.D.	Hot - water Bottles		Stationery
	and covers		Sweets
B.D.M.S.	Ice Bags		Sun Hats
	Jug Covers	O.D.	Shirts (Flannel)
	Kit Bags		„ (Cotton)
B.D.M.S.	Linen (Old for Ban-		„ Helpless Case
	dages)		„ Helpless Case
A.S.C.	Matches		(Night)
	Mirrors	O.D.	Screens
O.D.	Mosquito Netting	O.D.	Sheets
O.D.	Mugs, Enamelled	O.D.	Socks
O.D.	Mufflers		Sponges
	Mittens	O.D.	Slippers
	Nail Brushes	B.D.M.S.	Swabs
	Nightingales		Testaments
	Officers' Outfits	O.D.	Tooth Brushes
	Operation Stockings		Tooth Powder
O.D.	Overalls	A.S.C.	Tobacco
O.D.	Pants	O.D.	Towels
	Pencils	O.D.	Urinals
	Pipes		Vests
O.D.	Pillows		Walking Sticks
O.D.	Pillow Cases		Whisky
	Playing Cards		Wool, Absorbent
	Pneumonia Jackets	B.D.M.S.	Water Beds
	Post Cards	B.D.M.S.	Waterproof Sheeting
O.D.	Pyjamas		(Pluviusin)
O.D.	Razors		
	Razor Blades		*Extras*
	Reading Matter		
	Rum		

Items marked—

A.S.C.   (*Army Service Corps*),
O.D.   (*Ordnance Dept.*),
B.D.M.S.   (*Base Depot Medical Stores*),

will only be provided by the British Red Cross on the under-standing that the Military Departments have been applied to and cannot supply, or that it is a case of grave or unexpected emergency. Such a demand to be supported by signature of O.C. Hospital, which implies he has indented on the department concerned and failed to obtain.

N.B.—All indents to be countersigned by the O.C. Hospital.

The British Red Cross has definitely been placed under military control, and the chief commissioner has been attached to the staff of the commander-in-chief. The work goes on just as usual, but if necessity arose the commander-in-chief could exercise his authority.

I understand that in France the Australian Branch British Red Cross has now been placed under military control; the Director of Medical Services, Australian Expeditionary Force, being chief commissioner and the other commissioners and officers being graded with various ranks. To me this arrangement is definitely a step in the right direction, though I still think the British system in Egypt is better. The officers of the Red Cross in Egypt have no rank, but are under military direction, and the chief civil commissioner is attached to the staff of the commander-in-chief; he has had the rank of Hon. Colonel since the war began. It is interesting, however, to note that the Australian Branch British Red Cross has passed through four phases, so far as the work in the field is concerned:

(1) It was a purely military organisation.

(2) When the High Commissioner in Egypt was requested to form a committee it became a combined civil and military organisation.

(3) When the Australian commissioners were appointed it became a purely civil administration.

(4) It has finally become a combined civil and military organisation, in which the military element holds control.

This step further indicates the logical development, in my judgment, of both the Y.M.C.A. and the Red Cross. They should both be regarded as definite branches of the service. They should both be organised in time of peace largely as independent organisations, and as part of the Reserve, and, on declaration of war, they should be incorporated in the service and placed under military control. The function of the one would be to attend to the social wants of the men who are well, the other to attend to the wants of the men who are sick and wounded.

I do not think that any other funds or societies should be permitted to interfere with military arrangements; all those who desire to help with money, with goods, or with personal assistance could do so through the one channel or the other.

As a corollary to the foregoing it is evident that there should be only one voluntary war fund, which should be placed under the control of a committee representing the Y.M.C.A., the Red Cross, and nominees of the government and public, who could allocate the money subscribed to the Y.M.C.A. or Red Cross as necessity arose. The following list shows the unnecessary multiplicity of organisations and funds in the State of Victoria alone, *viz.* at least seventeen societies in a community of about one million and a half people.

Even in Egypt enthusiastic people started an "Australian Comforts Fund," a "Soldiers' Outings Association," "Camp Welfare Association," and so forth, and these bodies simply did for varying periods the work of the Y.M.C.A. or the Red Cross as the case may be, in a more or less patchy way.

MULTIPLICITY OF FUNDS

(From The Argus, Melbourne, 1916)

WAR RELIEF FUNDS

Objects Outlined: A Guide to Giving

It is only when one sees the complete list of war relief funds compiled by the State War Council, in connection with its announcement regarding the supervision to be exercised over future collections, that the full extent of the relief organisations and the wide scope covered by the Victorian public's generous giving are appreciated. There are in existence here a score of war funds of one kind or another, and by the devoted efforts of their organisers and the warm-hearted support of the public the lot of our soldiers has been brightened, the burden of pain and suffering borne by the sick and wounded has been eased, a helping hand has been extended to the homeless, broken sufferers of Belgium, Poland, and Serbia, and a gleam of happiness brought to many a home in France whose erstwhile breadwinner is on active service.

All the Victorian organisations have clearly defined objects, and are working along sound lines. The list of funds is to be increased shortly by the creation of a Repatriation Fund the details of which are now being worked out. The money raised will be devoted to the settling in suitable employment of soldiers who have fulfilled their service. A similar object is aimed at in the repatriation scheme which has been launched with such marked success by Mr. Rodgers, M.H.R. The objects of the other funds, which have been and are doing so much, are thus summarised for the information of the public by officials of the organisations:

British Red Cross Society
(Australian Branch)

Objects officially stated as—'Red Cross work, to assist all hospitals in time of war.'

Victorian Red Cross Fund

For Australian sick and wounded soldiers (Lady Stanley Appeal). The proceeds are being and will be remitted to the Australian Red Cross Society, to be used by it for the benefit of Australian sick and wounded soldiers and institutions in which they may be treated.

Red Cross Society
(Victorian Division)

Objects officially stated to be 'those of the Geneva Convention.'

French Red Cross Society

The raising of funds for the work of the French Red Cross Society.

Australian Patriotic Fund

For the benefit of Victorian soldiers and their dependents, soldiers from any part of Australia and their dependents, other deserving objects consequent on service at the war, and the augmenting of pensions granted by the Commonwealth.

State War Council's Fund

For discharged soldiers. Its object is to assist in re-establishing discharged soldiers in employment.

Commonwealth Button Fund

A collecting body, which has used its organisation for collecting for various funds. It has collected for the Belgian Fund, Red Cross Society, Lady Stanley's Appeal, French Red Cross, Serbian Fund, Italian Fund, Russian Polish Fund, and for institutions at the front and in camps belonging to the different churches and the Y.M.C.A.

Lady Mayoress's Patriotic League

To assist in providing comforts, extra clothing, and foods for the fighting men in the navy and army.

Belgian Relief Fund

To assist in relieving distress in Belgium.

Serbian Relief Fund
To assist in relieving distress amongst the Serbians.

Polish Relief Fund
To assist in relieving distress amongst the Russian Poles.

French Société Maternelle Fund
To collect funds for the *Société d'Assistance Maternelle et Infantile*. The fund is administered in France, money and goods being collected here and sent forward.

Y.M.C.A. National Appeal
For the benefit of soldiers in camps, on troopships, and abroad, by providing recreation, games, stationery, literature, and comforts, and ministering generally to the moral and spiritual welfare of the Australian troops.

Commonwealth Service Patriotic Fund
Objects determined, as necessity arises, by a committee consisting of heads of departments and branches. Allocations to different funds.

State Service Patriotic Fund
Relief of distress resulting from the war.

Education Department Patriotic Fund
Relief of distress caused by the war, and for providing clothing and comforts for our troops.

Railways Department Patriotic Fund
Relief of distress in Belgium, relief of distress due to unemployment in Victoria, and Red Cross purposes in the proportion as nearly as practicable of one-third to each.

An additional advantage of the arrangements proposed would be that all those who assist would be under a measure of discipline. Neither men nor women helpers should be permitted to enter the war zone unless they visit it with a serious purpose and an earnest desire to help. If they enter in this frame of mind they will have no objection to submitting to discipline. If they object it is far better for them to stay at home.

It is furthermore apparent that Red Cross workers should be limited to elderly men of experience or younger men who are physically defective. In the case of the Y.M.C.A. young and healthy men are required, since their work is very arduous, the living at times rough to a degree, and there is not inconsiderable personal risk undertaken by those who are placed in advanced positions. In national wars every healthy adult is of great value as a soldier, and it is necessary to see that as few of such men as possible are utilised in these auxiliary services.

If the arrangements here indicated had been carried into effect, the work in Egypt would have been much better done and the activities of the Y.M.C.A. would have prevented a vast amount of trouble and disease. As it was, the value of the Y.M.C.A. was not apparent to the public at first, since its activities are not so dramatic as those of the Red Cross Society, and funds have never been provided for it on anything like the same scale.

In conclusion, with regard to the Australian Branch British Red Cross, there is something more to be said. As its name implies, the Australian Red Cross is a branch of the British Red Cross Society, and yet we have experienced in Egypt the spectacle of the Egyptian Branch and the Australian Branch of the same society doing the same work for different sections of troops engaged in a common cause. There were two Red Cross stores in Cairo, Australian and British, two stores in Alexandria, and two in Mudros. Would it not have been much better to amalgamate the two branches and administer the Red Cross in Egypt as a whole? The separation served no good material purpose, and whilst by the exercise of good sense some of the difficulties arising from the dual arrangement were obviated, yet this evidence of particularism was not advantageous.

Vast quantities of goods were donated to the Australian Troops by the Comforts Fund, and vast quantities of goods were given to soldiers in hospitals and convalescent homes by the Australian Branch British Red Cross. As evidence of soundness of heart on the part of the Australian public this action was beyond praise, but it is doubtful whether the methods were the best which might be devised. The generosity of the public lent itself to some abuse, and soldiers are known to have sold these goods to Arabs, and employed the cash as they pleased. It is difficult to draw a healthy mean between strict administration with proper restriction and lavish administration and abuse.

It is doubtful to me whether it would not better conserve the self-respect of the soldier and be more dignified if these donations were to cease. In their place proper facilities might well be substituted for the purchase of such articles as the soldier required at very low prices. This is the plan followed by the Y.M.C.A., who never divorce personal service from any distribution of goods. If the pay of the Australian soldier—which by the way is the highest in the world—is thought insufficient, it could be increased by voluntary help conveyed through the proper official channels. If this system were adopted it would necessitate the appointment of a Y.M.C.A. and of a Red Cross officer to certain defined military units, and a well-organised method would at once make its appearance; in other words, we should substitute sympathetic order and justice for amateurish enthusiasm.

Does not the necessity for the foregoing criticism indicate our utter unpreparedness? For if we had possessed a national organisation for Peace and War, each and all of these problems would have been solved long ago, and we should have been spared the spectacle of willing helpers wasting their energy for lack of direction.

PREVENTION OF DISEASE

Surveying the whole campaign, the fundamental fault of the Australian Army Medical Service was the insufficient attention given to, and stress laid on, the prevention of disease. Is it not obvious that there should be a staff of medical officers and orderlies, detached altogether from any association with the treatment of disease, who should devote themselves entirely to the problem of prevention? This staff should be presided over by a surgeon-general who should be second only in rank to the Director of Medical Services in the field, and who with his staff should be armed with authority so far as the taking of steps for the prevention of disease is concerned.

At present the medical officers in the Australian Medical Service are entrusted with dual functions, the prevention and the treatment of disease.

So far there has been no Military School for medical officers in Australia, and until they are properly trained the prevention of disease will not be as effective as it might be.

In the Royal Army Medical Corps there is a Sanitary Staff, but it does not seem to me that even this highly trained body occupies the high position or enjoys the distinction that the value of its services really demand, and I cannot but think that it would be far better to abolish the term "sanitary" and to apply to it the term "Prophylactic Staff."

The cure of disease in civil life always attracts the public; it is dramatic and strikes the attention. The efforts of the men who obviate the necessity for anything of the kind never receive the same recognition, because the evil never becomes obvious.

Captain Lovegrove, A.A.M.C., was appointed Australian Embarkation Officer at Suez whilst I was in charge. He has contributed the following article to *The Australian Medical Journal* relative to the work he did during his ten months' stay.

MEDICAL NOTES ON TROOPS FROM AUSTRALIA LANDING AT SUEZ
By Frederick Lovegrove, M.B., Ch.B.(Melb.),
Captain A.A.M.C., Australia

During ten months' tenure of the unique appointment of Australian Embarkation Medical Officer, I have had peculiar opportunities of observing the condition of our soldiers arriving in Egypt.

The physique of our men has always excited the admiration of the British and Indian officers who have watched them disembark, and if an excess of high spirits in the troops has occasionally given an opportunity for military criticism, from a medical point of view this sign of robust health is altogether satisfactory.

The time of the voyage to Egypt from Melbourne averages thirty days; but, owing to delays at ports of call, many of the troops spend five weeks or more on board ship. The fact that the death-rate is so low and the condition of the men so good on arrival speaks highly for the arrangements on the ships and the watchful care of the medical officers on transport duty. A few accidents and an occasional case of appendicitis form the bulk of the cases removed to general wards of Suez Hospital.

Infectious disease, however, has occurred on a large number of vessels, and it has been possible to form some opinion of the epidemics present in the various camps in Australia, by noting the prevalent type of infectious disease on ships from different States.

(1) Influenza has been far and away the most common complaint. Though some of the patients are still febrile on arrival, and are sent to hospital here, the epidemic is usually spent before Egypt is reached.

(2) Pneumonia is occasionally severe, and is usually associated with an epidemic of influenza. Twelve months ago a certain percentage of cases developed empyema; for many months now

there have been no cases of this kind.

(3) Measles has been chiefly found among Victorian troops, and has been represented every month. South Australia has sent its quota during April and May. In some cases the epidemic has been wide-spread at first, and has worked itself out before arrival. In other cases a few men have been picked out early and isolated, and no epidemic has occurred. Occasionally a ship has arrived with a large number of cases, evidently originating after embarkation from some unrecognised case on board.

(4) Mumps has been represented largely every month. This disease is practically a perquisite of New South Wales and Queensland troops. The long incubation period and impossibility of recognising the disease in an early stage makes a general ship infection the rule, and the epidemic is usually at its height when the troops arrive here.

(5) Cerebro-spinal meningitis has not occurred as an epidemic, but has appeared on the returns every month, with one or two cases. Victoria has contributed the largest number of cases, except in November and January, when New South Wales supplied the largest number. Victoria has had a monopoly for the past four months.

(6) Enteric fever has been remarkable by its rarity. Ten cases only have been noted; of which New South Wales contributed six, five from one ship; Victoria one in each of the months of September, November, and December; and South Australia one in December. No cases have occurred this year.

"Chicken-pox, scarlet fever, and roetheln have occasioned no trouble here. Small-pox, plague, or cholera have not occurred among troops on Australian transports.

(7) Venereal disease. While the percentage of troops arriving in Egypt with venereal disease is not high—the actual figure is 0·75 *per cent.*—the total number of effectives withdrawn from combatant duty owing to this cause is sufficiently large to make the subject one of importance. In ten months 530 men with gonorrhœa and 90 men with syphilis have had to go to hospital immediately on arrival. Soft sores have almost always been cured on the voyage, so that practically all chancres seen here are syphilitic. By far the greatest number of syphilitic cases hail from Queensland and New South Wales, and while gonorrhœa is the main feature of Victorian venereal cases, the two previ-

ously mentioned States take the precedence here also.
A rise in the numbers from Western Australia has lately been noticed. This may possibly be due to the fact that men from other States found to be suffering from venereal diseases while crossing the Bight are landed in Western Australia. There is a general rise in the proportion of syphilis to gonorrhœa, and this is particularly noticeable among Queensland troops, where the general ratio of one syphilis to six gonorrhœa is now more like one to one, and occasionally the cases of gonorrhœa are outnumbered by syphilis.

Hospital Organisation

With extended experience the views of the writer on the subject of the organisation of military hospitals have crystallised. There is no doubt that the commander of a hospital must be a medical practitioner, and there is no doubt that in all matters relating to his hospital his authority must be final. In the last resort he must decide whether a patient is to leave the hospital or to stay; who should be admitted, and what the treatment should be. In a good organisation he will probably be very rarely required to express an opinion respecting these matters, but in the event of a conflict of opinion between say the consulting surgeon or physician and himself, there can be but one final arbitrament. The position is defined in the King's Regulations and is endorsed by common sense. So far as the registrar is concerned I think that he should be a medical practitioner, but that in every instance there should be an assistant registrar with the rank of lieutenant, who should do the whole of the detailed work connected with the records, and who need not necessarily be a medical officer. In like manner the transport officer and the orderly officer or adjutant should be of the same character and rank.

Difficulty, however, arises respecting the personnel of these non-medical offices. It is clear that, for purposes of discipline, they should belong to the Army Medical Corps and be under the control of the officer commanding. In time of war there is no doubt that invalided combatant officers would do very well, but no combatant officer would want such a position in time of peace, because there would be no subsequent career available. To effect a satisfactory solution of the problem it would be necessary to add to the establishment of a base hospital three non-medical commissioned officers of the same rank as the quartermaster, preferably former sergt.-majors who have obtained commissions and who consequently know the details of hospital administration thoroughly. There would then be in each base hospital four non-medical commissioned officers, *viz.* the quartermaster, the asst. registrar, the orderly officer, and the transport officer, and all would belong to the A.M.C. A hospital suitably staffed on this plan would run very smoothly.

ASSISTANCE OF ANGLO-EGYPTIANS

Surveying the work of the Australian Army Medical Corps in Egypt, it does seem to me that sufficient acknowledgment has not been made of the services rendered and the help given to the Australian sick and wounded by the British residents in Egypt, who, from their Excellencies Sir Henry and Lady MacMahon downwards, spared no effort to help wherever assistance was possible. Very many of the officials employed in the Egyptian Government service came to the hospitals when the day's work was over and worked till late in the night, rendering services which freed the orderlies for other special duty. It was impossible to get reinforcements with any rapidity, the pressure was enormous, and the least that can be said is that these ladies and gentlemen are entitled to respectful and grateful acknowledgment from the people of Australia.

Special acknowledgment also should be made of the sympathetic help given by the courteous and able officers of the Egyptian State Railways.

I do not think it will be right to close the work without personal acknowledgment of the exceedingly valuable help given in a time of crisis by the ladies and gentlemen whose names are attached, and who, at great inconvenience, came forward at the time when other help was unobtainable.

No. 1 AUSTRALIAN GENERAL HOSPITAL—HELIOPOLIS PALACE

From its establishment until the opening of No. 2 General Hospital

Principal Red Cross Visitor

Mrs. Elgood

Ward Visitors (daily or several times a week)

Lady Oakes	The Hon. Mrs. Home
Mrs. Abramson	Lady Cheetham
Mrs. Blakeney	Mrs. Everett
Mrs. Frank Watson	Miss Devonshire
Mrs. Boys	Mrs. Teal
Mrs. Madden	Lady Douglas
Lady Brunyate	Mrs. Paxton
Mrs. Perels	Mrs. Fletcher
Mrs. Dale	Mrs. Dunhill
Mrs. Mackworth	

Most valuable assistance was also rendered by Mrs. Travers Symons and Mrs. W. Jessop.

Flower Ladies (visiting three times a week)

Mrs. Hodgson	Mrs. Garrett
Mrs. Spong	Mrs. Spencer Smith
Miss Marshall	Mrs. Lumley Smith
Mrs. Crawley	

HELIOPOLIS

From the opening of the No. 2 General Hospital, till end of July 1915

Principal Visitor

Mrs. Elgood

Ward Visitors (daily or several times a week)

Lady Oakes	Mrs. Fletcher
Mrs. Waller	Mrs. Spencer Smith
Mrs. Sender	Mrs. Dawnay
Mrs. Fox	Mrs. and Miss Knox
Mrs. Summons	Mrs. and the Misses Spens
Mrs. Maxwell	Three Ladies from C.M.S.
Miss Mavris	Mme. and Mlle. de Lancker
Mr. Dulle	Mme. de Rey
Mr. Schreiber	Mrs. Dunbar Brunton
Major Blakeney	Miss Hanauer
Mrs. Blakeney	Mrs. Watson
Mrs. MacDonald	Mr. St. Clair
Mrs. Everett	Dr. Grace Russell

187

Mrs. H. Chisholme
The Hon. Mrs. Home
Mrs. Perels
Mrs. Dale

Mrs. Adie
Mrs. Wisdom
Mrs. Makeham
Mrs. Bruce.

Organiser of Concerts

The Countess de Lavison

No. 1 AUSTRALIAN GENERAL HOSPITAL

Gentlemen who did Telephone Duty at Heliopolis Palace

Mr. H. O. Bennett, Kubba Gardens
Mr. G. Brackenbury, late of Palais de Kubba
Mr. L. Billson, Zeitoun
Mr. N. L. Ablett, Helmieh
Mr. A. Abramson, late of Heliopolis
Mr. T. H. Clarke, Zeitoun
Mr. G. R. Tadman, late of Heliopolis
Mr. H. B. May, late of Zeitoun
Mr. A. R. B. Milton, Heliopolis
Mr. S. Fraser, Heliopolis.
Mr. R. Lawson, Heliopolis.
Mr. M. R. Pattison, Zeitoun.
Mr. G. Muller, Kafr el Gamous
Mr. H. E. Gardiner, Kafr el Gamous
Mr. E. Griffith Jones, Mataria
Mr. J. C. Mansfield, Kubba les Bains.
Mr. J. K. Parkes, late of Heliopolis.
Mr. Hanauer (Senr.), late of Heliopolis.

LUNA PARK—SKATING RINK

From opening till middle of July 1915

Principal Visitor

Lady Oakes

Ward Visitors (daily or several times a week)

Mrs. Spencer Smith
Mrs. Elgood
Mrs. H. Chisholme
Miss Griffiths
Mrs. Wellburn
Mrs. Barry Davies
The Misses Crewe (2)
Mrs. Woodifield
Mrs. Clogstoun
Mrs. Mackworth
Major Blakeney
Mrs. Teasdale Smith
Mrs. Rebett

Miss Christian
Mrs. Knox
Mrs. Parlato
Mme. Yenidimia
Mrs. Bailey
Mrs. Everett
Mrs. Williams
Mr. Blythe
Mrs. Makeham
Mrs. Bruce
Mr. Naggiar
Mr. Airlet
Mrs. Fenwick

Daily Ward Workers

Miss Villedieu	Mrs. Sender
Mrs. Addison	Mrs. Walker
Miss Ratzkowski	Mrs. Fox
Mrs. Le Fleming	Miss Morrison
Mrs. Murray	Miss Pound
The Hon Mrs. Morrison Bell	Mrs. Wilson
Mrs. Hibbert	Mlle. Picciotti
Mrs. and Miss Leathes	Mrs. Fanous

LUNA PARK PAVILION

Principal Visitor

Mr. Blythe

Helpers

Mr. and Mrs. May, late of Zeitoun
Mr. and Mrs. Bennett, Kubba Gardens
Mr. and Mrs. Micklam, Palais Kubba
Mr. and Mrs. Stopford, Zeitoun
Mr. and Mrs. Ablett, Helmieh
Mr. and Mrs. Levy, Heliopolis.
Mr. and Mrs. Hood, late of Kubba Gardens
Mr. and Mrs. Clarke, now at Kubba les Bains
Mrs. T. and Miss Williams, Zeitoun
Mrs. Watkins, late of Zeitoun
Mrs. Hogan, late of Zeitoun
Mrs. Fenwick, Helmieh
Mrs. Tite, Zeitoun
Mr. Goadby, late of Zeitoun
Mr. Brackenbury, late of Palais Kubba
Mr. Poths, now at Kubba les Bains

ATELIER

Principal Visitor

Mr. Goadby

Daily Workers

Mrs. Goadby	Mrs. Dawnay (*Librarian*)
Mrs. and the Misses Spens	Mrs. Morris

SPORTING CLUB

Principal Visitor

Mr. Herbert

Daily Worker

Mrs. Eddy (after Nov. 1916)

[The first Inquiry Bureau in Egypt for service in connection with the Wounded and Missing was established by Mrs. Jessop, of the Y.M.C.A.]

Appendix 1: Translation of Geneva Convention of July 6, 1906

Article 1

Officers and soldiers, and other persons officially attached to armies, shall be respected and taken care of when wounded or sick by the belligerent in whose power they may be, without distinction of nationality.

Nevertheless, a belligerent who is compelled to abandon sick or wounded to the enemy shall, as far as military exigencies permit, leave with them a portion of his medical *personnel* and material to contribute to the care of them.

Article 2

Except as regards the treatment to be provided for them in virtue of the preceding article, the wounded and sick of an army who fall into the hands of an enemy are prisoners of war, and the general provisions of international law concerning prisoners are applicable to them.

Belligerents are, however, free to arrange with one another such exceptions and mitigations with reference to sick and wounded prisoners as they may judge expedient; in particular, they will be at liberty to agree—

To restore to one another the wounded left on the field after a battle;

To repatriate any wounded and sick whom they do not wish to retain as prisoners, after rendering them fit for removal or after recovery;

To hand over to a neutral State, with the latter's consent, the enemy's wounded and sick to be interned by the neutral State until the end of hostilities.

Article 3

After each engagement the commander in possession of the field shall take measures to search for the wounded, and to ensure protection against pillage and maltreatment both for the wounded and for the dead.

He shall arrange that a careful examination of the bodies is made before the dead are buried or cremated.

Article 4

As early as possible each belligerent shall send to the authorities of the country or army to which they belong the military identification marks or tokens found on the dead, and a nominal roll of the wounded or sick who have been collected by him.

The belligerents shall keep each other mutually informed of any internments and changes, as well as of admissions into hospital and deaths among the wounded and sick in their hands. They shall collect all the articles of personal use, valuables, letters, etc., which are found on the field of battle or left by the wounded or sick who have died in the medical establishments or units, in order that such objects may be transmitted to the persons interested by the authorities of their own country.

Article 5

The competent military authority may appeal to the charitable zeal of the inhabitants to collect and take care of, under his direction, the wounded or sick of armies, granting to those who respond to the appeal special protection and certain immunities.

CHAPTER 2
MEDICAL UNITS AND ESTABLISHMENTS

Article 6

Mobile medical units (that is to say, those which are intended to accompany armies into the field) and the fixed establishments of the medical service shall be respected and protected by the belligerents.

Article 7

The protection to which medical units and establishments are entitled ceases if they are made use of to commit acts harmful to the enemy.

Article 8

The following facts are not considered to be of a nature to deprive a medical unit or establishment of the protection guaranteed by Article 6:—

1. That the *personnel* of the unit or of the establishment is armed, and that it uses its arms for its own defence or for that of the sick and wounded under its charge.

2. That in default of armed orderlies the unit or establishment is guarded by a picquet or by sentinels furnished with an authority in due form.

3. That weapons and cartridges taken from the wounded and not yet handed over to the proper department are found in the unit or establishment.

Chapter 3
Personnel
Article 9

The *personnel* engaged exclusively in the collection, transport, and treatment of the wounded and the sick, as well as in the administration of medical units and establishments, and the chaplains attached to armies, shall be respected and protected under all circumstances. If they fall into the hands of the enemy they shall not be treated as prisoners of war.

These provisions apply to the guard of medical units and establishments under the circumstances indicated in Article 8 (2).

Article 10

The *personnel* of Voluntary Aid Societies, duly recognised and authorised by their government, who may be employed in the medical units and establishments of armies, is placed on the same footing as the *personnel* referred to in the preceding article, provided always that the first-mentioned *personnel* shall be subject to military law and regulations.

Each State shall notify to the other, either in time of peace or at the commencement of or during the course of hostilities, but in every case before actually employing them, the names of the societies which it has authorised, under its responsibility, to render assistance to the regular medical service of its armies.

Article 11

A recognised society of a neutral country can only afford the assistance of its medical *personnel* and units to a belligerent with the previous consent of its own government and the authorisation of the belligerent concerned.

A belligerent who accepts such assistance is bound to notify the fact to his adversary before making any use of it.

Article 12

The persons designated in Articles 9, 10, and 11, after they have fallen into the hands of the enemy, shall continue to carry on their duties under his direction.

When their assistance is no longer indispensable, they shall be sent back to their army or to their country at such time and by such route as may be compatible with military exigencies.

They shall then take with them such effects, instruments, arms, and horses as are their private property.

Article 13

The enemy shall secure to the persons mentioned in Article 9, while in his hands, the same allowances and the same pay as are granted to the persons holding the same rank in his own army.

CHAPTER 4

MATERIAL

Article 14

If mobile medical units fall into the hands of the enemy they shall retain their material, including their teams, irrespectively of the means of transport and the drivers employed.

Nevertheless, the competent military authority shall be free to use the material for the treatment of the wounded and sick. It shall be restored under the conditions laid down for the medical *personnel*, and so far as possible at the same time.

Article 15

The buildings and material of fixed establishments remain subject to the laws of war, but may not be diverted from their purpose so long as they are necessary for the wounded and the sick.

Nevertheless, the commanders of troops in the field may dispose of them, in case of urgent military necessity, provided they make previous arrangements for the welfare of the wounded and sick who are found there.

Article 16

The material of Voluntary Aid Societies which are admitted to the privileges of the Convention under the conditions laid down therein is considered private property, and as such to be respected under all circumstances, saving only the right of requisition recognised for belligerents in accordance with the laws and customs of war.

CHAPTER 5
CONVOYS OF EVACUATION
Article 17

Convoys of evacuation shall be treated like mobile medical units subject to the following special provisions:—

1. A belligerent intercepting a convoy may break it up if military exigencies demand, provided he takes charge of the sick and wounded who are in it.

2. In this case, the obligation to send back the medical *personnel*, provided for in Article 12, shall be extended to the whole of the military *personnel* detailed for the transport or the protection of the convoy, and furnished with an authority in due form to that effect.

The obligation to restore the medical material, provided for in Article 14, shall apply to railway trains, and boats used in internal navigation, which are specially arranged for evacuations, as well as to the material belonging to the medical service for fitting up ordinary vehicles, trains, and boats.

Military vehicles other than those of the medical service may be captured with their teams.

The civilian *personnel* and the various means of transport obtained by requisition, including railway material and boats used for convoys, shall be subject to the general rules of international law.

CHAPTER 6
THE DISTINCTIVE EMBLEM
Article 18

As a compliment to Switzerland, the heraldic emblem of the red cross on a white ground, formed by reversing the Federal colours, is retained as the emblem and distinctive sign of the medical service of armies.

Article 19

With the permission of the competent military authority, this emblem shall be shown on the flags and armlets (*brassards*), as well as on all the material belonging to the Medical Service.

Article 20

The *personnel* protected in pursuance of Articles 9 (paragraph 1), 10, and 11 shall wear, fixed to the left arm, an armlet (*brassard*), with a red cross on a white ground, delivered and stamped by the competent military authority, and accompanied by a certificate of identity in the case of persons who are attached to the medical service of armies, but who have not a military uniform.

Article 21

The distinctive flag of the Convention shall only be hoisted over those medical units and establishments which are entitled to be respected under the Convention, and with the consent of the military authorities. It must be accompanied by the national flag of the belligerent to whom the unit or establishment belongs.

Nevertheless, medical units which have fallen into the hands of the enemy, so long as they are in that situation, shall not fly any other flag than that of the Red Cross.

Article 22

The medical units belonging to neutral countries which may be authorised to afford their services under the conditions laid down in Article 11 shall fly, along with the flag of the Convention, the national flag of the belligerent to whose army they are attached.

The provisions of the second paragraph of the preceding article are applicable to them.

Article 23

The emblem of the red cross on a white ground and the words "Red Cross" or "Geneva Cross" shall not be used either in time of peace or in time of war, except to protect or to indicate the medical units and establishments and the *personnel* and material protected by the Convention.

CHAPTER 7

APPLICATION AND CARRYING OUT OF THE CONVENTION

Article 24

The provisions of the present Convention are only binding upon the Contracting Powers in the case of war between two or more of them. These provisions shall cease to be binding from the moment when one of the belligerent Powers is not a party to the Convention.

Article 25

The commanders-in-chief of belligerent armies shall arrange the details for carrying out the preceding articles, as well as for cases not provided for, in accordance with the instructions of their respective governments, and in conformity with the general principles of the present Convention.

Article 26

The Signatory Governments will take the necessary measures to instruct their troops, especially the *personnel* protected, in the provisions of the present Convention, and to bring them to the notice of the civil population.

CHAPTER 8
PREVENTION OF ABUSES AND INFRACTIONS
Article 27

The Signatory Governments, in countries the legislation of which is not at present adequate for the purpose, undertake to adopt or to propose to their legislative bodies such measures as may be necessary to prevent at all times the employment of the emblem or the name of Red Cross or Geneva Cross by private individuals or by societies other than those which are entitled to do so under the present Convention, and in particular for commercial purposes as a trade-mark or trading mark.

The prohibition of the employment of the emblem or the names in question shall come into operation from the date fixed by each legislature, and at the latest five years after the present Convention comes into force. From that date it shall no longer be lawful to adopt a trade-mark or trading mark contrary to this prohibition.

Article 28

The Signatory Governments also undertake to adopt, or to propose to their legislative bodies, should their military law be insufficient for the purpose, the measures necessary for the repression in time of war of individual acts of pillage and maltreatment of the wounded and sick of armies, as well as for the punishment, as an unlawful employment of military insignia, of the improper use of the Red Cross flag and armlet (*brassard*) by officers and soldiers or private individuals not protected by the present Convention.

They shall communicate to one another, through the Swiss Federal Council, the provisions relative to these measures of repression at the latest within five years from the ratification of the present Convention.

GENERAL PROVISIONS
Article 29

The present Convention shall be ratified as soon as possible. The ratifications shall be deposited at Berne.

When each ratification is deposited a *procès verbal* shall be drawn up, and a copy thereof certified as correct shall be forwarded through the diplomatic channel to all the Contracting Powers.

Article 30

The present Convention shall come into force for each Power six months after the date of the deposit of its ratification.

Article 31

The present Convention, duly ratified, shall replace the Convention of August 22nd, 1864, in relations between the Contracting States. The Convention of 1864 remains in force between such of the parties who signed it who may not likewise ratify the present Convention.

Article 32

The present Convention may be signed until December 31st next by the Powers represented at the Conference, which was opened at Geneva on June 11, 1906, as also by the Powers, not represented at that Conference, which signed the Convention of 1864.

Such of the aforesaid Powers as shall have not signed the present Convention by December 31st, 1906, shall remain free to accede to it subsequently. They shall notify their accession by means of a written communication addressed to the Swiss Federal Council, and communicated by the latter to all the Contracting Powers.

Other Powers may apply to accede in the same manner, but their request shall only take effect if within a period of one year from the notification of it to the Federal Council no objection to it reaches the Council from any of the Contracting Powers.

Article 33

Each of the Contracting Powers shall be at liberty to denounce the present Convention. The denunciation shall not take effect until one year after the written notification of it has reached the Swiss Federal Council. The council shall immediately communicate the notification to all the other Contracting Parties.

The denunciation shall only affect the Power which has notified it.

Appendix 2: Convention for the Adaptation of the Principles of the Geneva Convention to Maritime War

His Majesty the German Emperor, King of Prussia; the President of the United States of America; the President of the Argentine Republic; His Majesty the Emperor of Austria, King of Bohemia, etc., and Apostolic King of Hungary; His Majesty the King of the Belgians; the President of the Republic of Bolivia; the President of the Republic of the United States of Brazil; His Royal Highness the Prince of Bulgaria; the President of the Republic of Chile; His Majesty the Emperor of China; the President of the Republic of Colombia; the Provisional Governor of the Republic of Cuba; His Majesty the King of Denmark; the President of the Dominican Republic; the President of the Republic of Ecuador; His Majesty the King of Spain; the President of the French Republic; His Majesty the King of the United Kingdom of Great Britain and Ireland and of the British Dominions beyond the Seas, Emperor of India; His Majesty the King of the Hellenes; the President of the Republic of Guatemala; the President of the Republic of Haiti; His Majesty the King of Italy; His Majesty the Emperor of Japan; His Royal Highness the Grand Duke of Luxemburg, Duke of Nassau; the President of the United States of Mexico; His Royal Highness the Prince of Montenegro; the President of the Republic of Nicaragua; His Majesty the King of Norway; the President of the Republic of Panama; the President of the Republic of Paraguay; Her Majesty the Queen of the Netherlands; the President of the Republic of Peru; His Imperial Majesty the Shah of Persia; His Majesty the King of Portugal and of the Algarves, etc.; His Majesty the King of Roumania; His Majesty the Emperor of All the Russias; the

President of the Republic of Salvador; His Majesty the King of Serbia; His Majesty the King of Siam; His Majesty the King of Sweden; the Swiss Federal Council; His Majesty the Emperor of the Ottomans; the President of the Oriental Republic of Uruguay; the President of the United States of Venezuela:

Animated alike by the desire to diminish, as far as depends on them, the inevitable evils of war; and

Wishing with this object to adapt to maritime war the principles of the Geneva Convention of July 6, 1906:

Have resolved to conclude a Convention for the purpose of revising the Convention of July 29, 1899, relative to this question, and have appointed as their Plenipotentiaries, that is to say:

(Names of Plenipotentiaries.)

Who, after having deposited their full powers, found to be in good and due form, have agreed upon the following provisions:—

Article 1

Military hospital-ships, that is to say, ships constructed or adapted by States for the particular and sole purpose of aiding the sick, wounded, and shipwrecked, the names of which have been communicated to the belligerent Powers at the commencement or during the course of hostilities, and in any case before they are employed, shall be respected, and may not be captured while hostilities last.

Such ships, moreover, are not on the same footing as war-ships as regards their stay in a neutral port.

Article 2

Hospital-ships, equipped wholly or in part at the expense of private individuals or officially recognised relief societies, shall likewise be respected and exempt from capture, if the belligerent Power to which they belong has given them an official commission and has notified their names to the hostile Power at the commencement of or during hostilities, and in any case before they are employed.

Such ships shall be provided with a certificate from the proper authorities declaring that the vessels have been under their control while fitting out and on final departure.

Article 3

Hospital-ships, equipped wholly or in part at the expense of private individuals or officially recognised societies of neutral countries, shall be respected and exempt from capture, on condition that they are placed under the orders of one of the belligerents, with the previous consent of their own government and with the authorisation of the belligerent himself, and on condition also that the latter has notified their name to his adversary at the commencement of or during hostilities, and in any case before they are employed.

Article 4

The ships mentioned in Articles 1, 2, and 3 shall afford relief and assistance to the wounded, sick, and shipwrecked of the belligerents without distinction of nationality.

The governments undertake not to use these ships for any military purpose.

Such vessels must in no wise hamper the movements of the combatants.

During and after an engagement they will act at their own risk and peril.

The belligerents shall have the right to control and search them; they may refuse to help them, order them off, make them take a certain course, and put a commissioner on board; they may even detain them, if the situation is such as to require it.

The belligerents shall, as far as possible, enter in the log of the hospital-ships the orders which they give them.

Article 5

Military hospital-ships shall be distinguished by being painted white outside with a horizontal band of green about a metre and a half in breadth.

The ships mentioned in Articles 2 and 3 shall be distinguished by being painted white outside with a horizontal band of red about a metre and a half in breadth.

The boats of the said ships, as also small craft which may be used for hospital work, shall be distinguished by similar painting.

All hospital-ships shall make themselves known by hoisting, with their national flag, the white flag with a red cross provided by the Geneva Convention, and further, if they belong to a neutral State, by flying at the mainmast the national flag of the belligerent under whose orders they are placed.

Hospital-ships which are detained under Article 4 by the enemy must haul down the national flag of the belligerent to whom they belong.

The ships and boats above mentioned which wish to ensure by night the freedom from interference to which they are entitled, must, subject to the assent of the belligerent they are accompanying, take the necessary measures to render their special painting sufficiently plain.

Article 6

The distinguishing signs referred to in Article 5 shall only be used, whether in peace or war, for protecting or indicating the ships therein mentioned.

Article 7

In the case of a fight on board a war-ship, the sick-bays shall be respected and spared as far as possible.

The said sick-bays and the *matériel* belonging to them remain subject to the laws of war; they cannot, however, be used for any purpose other than that for which they were originally intended, so long as they are required for the sick and wounded.

The commander into whose power they have fallen may, however, if the military situation requires it, apply them to other purposes, after seeing that the sick and wounded on board are properly provided for.

Article 8

Hospital-ships and sick-bays of vessels are no longer entitled to protection if they are employed for the purpose of injuring the enemy.

The fact of the staff of the said ships and sick-bays being armed for maintaining order and for defending the sick and wounded, and the presence of wireless telegraphy apparatus on board, are not sufficient reasons for withdrawing protection.

Article 9

Belligerents may appeal to the charity of the commanders of neutral merchant-ships, yachts, or boats to take the sick and wounded on board and tend them.

Vessels responding to this appeal, and also vessels which may have of their own accord rescued sick, wounded, or shipwrecked men, shall enjoy special protection and certain immunities. In no case may they be captured for the sole reason of having such persons on board; but, subject to any undertaking that may have been given to them, they remain liable to capture for any violations of neutrality they may have committed.

Article 10

The religious, medical, and hospital staff of any captured ship is inviolable, and its members may not be made prisoners of war. On leaving the ship they are entitled to remove their own private belongings and surgical instruments.

They shall continue to discharge their duties so far as necessary, and can afterwards leave, when the commander-in-chief considers it permissible.

Belligerents must guarantee to the said staff, while in their hands, the same allowances and pay as are given to the staff of corresponding rank in their own navy.

Article 11

Sick or wounded sailors, soldiers on board, or other persons officially attached to fleets or armies, whatever their nationality, shall be respected and tended by the captors.

Article 12

Any war-ship belonging to a belligerent may demand the surrender of sick, wounded, or shipwrecked men on board military hospital-ships, hospital-ships belonging to relief societies or to private individuals, merchant-ships, yachts, or boats, whatever the nationality of such vessels.

Article 13

If sick, wounded, or shipwrecked persons are taken on board a neutral war-ship, precaution must be taken, so far as possible, that they do not again take part in the operations of the war.

Article 14

The sick, wounded, or shipwrecked of one of the belligerents who fall into the power of the other belligerent are prisoners of war. The captor must decide, according to circumstances, whether to keep them, send them to a port of his own country, to a neutral port, or even to an enemy port. In this last case, prisoners thus repatriated may not serve again while the war lasts.

Article 15

The sick, wounded, or shipwrecked, who are landed at a neutral port with the consent of the local authorities, must, in default of arrangement to the contrary between the neutral State and the belligerent States, be guarded by the neutral States so as to prevent them from again taking part in the operations of the war.

The expenses of tending them in hospital and interning them shall be borne by the State to which the shipwrecked, sick, or wounded persons belong.

Article 16

After every engagement, the two belligerents shall, so far as military interests permit, take steps to look for the sick, wounded, and shipwrecked, and to protect them, as well as the dead, against pillage and improper treatment.

They shall see that the burial, whether by land or sea, or cremation of the dead shall be preceded by a careful examination of the corpse.

Article 17

Each belligerent shall send, as early as possible, the military marks or documents of identity found on the dead and a list of the names of the sick and wounded picked up by him to the authorities of their country, navy, or army.

The belligerents shall keep each other informed as to internments and transfers as well as to the admissions into hospital and deaths which have occurred among the sick and wounded in their hands. They shall collect all the objects of personal use, valuables, letters, etc., which may be found in the captured ships, or which may have been left by the sick or wounded who died in hospital, in order to have them forwarded to the persons concerned by the authorities of their own country.

Article 18

The provisions of the present Convention do not apply except between Contracting Powers, and then only if all the belligerents are parties to the Convention.

Article 19

The commander-in-chief of the belligerent fleets shall give detailed directions for carrying out the preceding Articles and for meeting cases not therein provided for, in accordance with the instructions of their respective governments and in conformity with the general principles of the present Convention.

Article 20

The Signatory Powers shall take the necessary steps in order to bring the provisions of the present Convention to the knowledge of their naval forces, and especially of the members entitled thereunder to immunity, and to make them known to the public.

Article 21

The Signatory Powers likewise undertake to enact or to propose to their legislatures, if their criminal laws are inadequate, the measures necessary for checking in time of war individual acts of pillage and ill-treatment in respect to the sick and wounded in the fleet, as well as for punishing as an unjustifiable adoption of naval or military marks, the unauthorised use of the distinctive marks mentioned in Article 5, by vessels not protected by the present Convention.

They shall communicate to each other, through the Netherland Government, the enactments for preventing such acts at the latest within five years of the ratification of the present Convention.

Article 22

In the case of operations of war between the land and sea forces of belligerents, the provisions of the present Convention are only applicable to the forces on board ship.

Article 23

The present Convention shall be ratified as soon as possible.

The ratifications shall be deposited at The Hague.

The first deposit of ratifications shall be recorded in a protocol signed by the Representatives of the Powers which take part therein and by the Netherland Minister for Foreign Affairs.

The subsequent deposits of ratifications shall be made by means of a written notification, addressed to the Netherland Government and accompanied by the instrument of ratification.

A duly certified copy of the protocol relating to the first deposit of ratifications, of the notifications mentioned in the preceding paragraph, and of the instruments of ratification, shall be immediately sent by the Netherland Government through the diplomatic channel to the Powers invited to the Second Peace Conference, as well as to the other Powers which have acceded to the Convention. The said government shall, in the cases contemplated in the preceding paragraph, inform them at the same time of the date on which it received the notification.

Article 24

Non-Signatory Powers which have accepted the Geneva Convention of July 6, 1906, may accede to the present Convention.

A Power which desires to accede notifies its intention in writing to the Netherland Government, forwarding to it the act of accession, which shall be deposited in the archives of the said government.

The said government shall immediately forward to all the other Powers a duly certified copy of the notification, as well as of the act of accession, mentioning the date on which it received the notification.

Article 25

The present Convention, duly ratified, shall replace, as between Contracting Powers, the Convention of July 29, 1899, for the adaptation to naval warfare of the principles of the Geneva Convention.

The Convention of 1899 remains in force as between the Powers which signed it but which do not also ratify the present Convention.

Article 26

The present Convention shall take effect, in the case of the Powers which were parties to the first deposit of ratifications, sixty days after the date of the protocol recording such deposit, and, in the case of the Powers which shall ratify subsequently or which shall accede, sixty days after the notification of their ratification or of their accession has been received by the Netherland Government.

Article 27

In the event of one of the Contracting Powers wishing to denounce the present Convention, the denunciation shall be notified in writing to the Netherland Government, which shall immediately communicate a duly certified copy of the notification to all the other Powers, informing them of the date on which it was received.

The denunciation shall only operate in respect of the denouncing Power, and only on the expiry of one year after the notification has reached the Netherland Government.

Article 28

A register kept by the Netherland Ministry for Foreign Affairs shall record the date of the deposit of ratifications effected in virtue of Article 23, paragraphs 3 and 4, as well as the date on which the notifications of accession (Article 24, paragraph 2) or of denunciation (Article 27, paragraph 1) have been received.

Each Contracting Power is entitled to have access to this register and to be supplied with duly certified extracts from it.

In faith whereof the plenipotentiaries have appended their signatures to the present Convention.

Done at The Hague, October 18, 1907, in a single original, which shall remain deposited in the archives of the Netherland Government, and of which duly certified copies shall be sent, through the diplomatic channel, to the Powers invited to the Second Peace Conference.

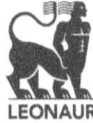